REHABILITATION PROTOCOLS FOR SURGICAL AND NONSURGICAL PROCEDURES

LUMBAR SPINE

REHABILITATION PROTOCOLS FOR SURGICAL AND NONSURGICAL PROCEDURES

Lumbar Spine

CAROL M. McFARLAND P.T, M.S., O.C.S.
DON H. BURKHART, P.T.

Preface by Aubrey A. Swartz, M.D., Pharm.D.
Foreword by Philip E. Greenman, D.O., F.A.A.O.

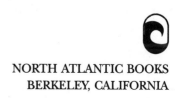

NORTH ATLANTIC BOOKS
BERKELEY, CALIFORNIA

Published by

North Atlantic Books   Cover and book design by Jan Camp
P.O. Box 12327
Berkeley, California 94712   Printed in the United States of America

Rehabilitation Protocols for Surgical and Nonsurgical Procedures: Lumbar Spine is sponsored by the Society for the Study of Native Arts and Sciences, a nonprofit educational corporation whose goals are to develop an educational and crosscultural perspective linking various scientific, social, and artistic fields; to nurture a holistic view of arts, sciences, humanities, and healing; and to publish and distribute literature on the relationship of mind, body, and nature.

North Atlantic Books' publications are available through most bookstores. For further information, call 800-337-2665 or visit our website at www.northatlanticbooks.com.

Substantial discounts on bulk quantities are available to corporations, professional associations, and other organizations. For details and discount information, contact our special sales department.

Library of Congress Cataloging-in-Publication Data

McFarland, Carol.
    Rehabilitation Protocols for Surgical and Nonsurgical Procedures: Lumbar Spine / Carol McFarland and Don H. Burkhart.
        p. cm.
    Includes bibliographical references.
        ISBN 1-55643-380-8 (alk. paper)
        1. Lumbar vertebrae—Wounds and injuries—Diagnosis—Handbooks, manuals, etc. 2. Spine—Surgery—Handbooks, manuals, etc. 3. Spine—Wounds and injuries—Patients—Rehabilitation—Handbooks, manuals, etc. 4. Spine—Wounds and injuries—Physical Therapy—Handbooks, manuals, etc.
    I. Burkhart, Don H.II. Title.
    RD768 .M39 2001
    617.5'6—dc21   2001030941
                                                                CIP

        1 2 3 4 5 6 7 8 9 / 06 05 04 03 02 01

To my husband Tom, who is always right there helping me look for the pony, and to my whole family, a great source of joy in my life.

—C.M.M.

To the hundreds of physical therapists, physicians, and educators who have inspired us throughout the years and have paved the way for us to complete a project like this one.

—D.H.B. and C.M.M.

Contents

List of Figures

Foreword

The health care system continues to deal with a plethora of patients who present with low back pain: acute, chronic and recurrent. These patients use many valuable resources in the system and the cost to society is large. However, to date there is no consensus on cause or treatment of these patients. New information is added to old as we learn more about this enigmatic problem, and it has not been organized and presented in a systematic manner.

Physical therapy, as part of the rehabilitation of patients with low back pain, has much support in the health care system and many methods are used. This well-designed text provides both the physical therapist and the referring physician information of great value for treating both the surgical and non-surgical patient. In easily readable form, it presents basic principles of the rehabilitative process and provides usable specific protocols for physical therapy. It combines information from many different authors and teachers of physical therapy in a well-organized manner that gives good direction for the neophyte and the expert. Included are many record forms for use in the original assessment of the patient and for continuing record of progress. Fundamental exercises for patient use are also included.

This volume is a valuable addition to the library of the spine care practitioner.

—Philip E. Greenman, D.O., F.A.A.O.
Professor Emeritus, Physical Medicine and Rehabilitation and
Osteopathic Manipulative Medicine, Michigan State University,
President American Back Society 2000

Preface

The field of spinal care has been changing and making a great deal of progress over the past several years. Advances in physical therapy and rehabilitative methods and techniques have been in the forefront of this remarkable progress, and the contributions by physical therapists have made a great deal of difference in the quality of health care delivery to patients with spinal afflictions. Carol McFarland, Don Burkhart, and Guy Danielson have taken their place alongside the leaders in the field of spinal care, with the recognized support of their outstanding colleagues at NeuroCare Network and the East Texas Neurological Institute. The authors of this book have compiled the results of this group's efforts to make the work with spinal patients systematic.

Rehabilitation following spine surgery is an essential part of treatment. The authors have gathered scientific data over several years supporting this very important concept. The authors rightfully emphasize the critical need for overcoming chronic dysfunction, deconditioning, and anatomic changes resulting from many surgical procedures. Emphasis on the functional improvement of the patient is clearly demonstrated in this book, and it is restoring function that is the ultimate goal of the physical therapist. The authors provide excellent comprehensive discussions on the preoperative examination and evaluation of the spine patient, evaluation of the postoperative patient, differentiating the physical therapy protocols that would be most appropriate for each type of surgical and spinal injection procedure. They have supported their methods with appropriate scientific references, and thus this book should provide information to research and customize specific rehabilitation protocols for practitioners in their own particular spine care facilities.

—Aubrey A. Swartz, M.D., Pharm. D.
Executive Director, American Back Society

Acknowledgments

This book is the result of an eight-year effort inspired by Guy O. Danielson, M.D., an innovative neurosurgeon who has always explored all possibilities for the best care of his patients. Due to the many spine patients referred by Dr. Danielson and the reputation he has helped us achieve as spine specialists, we have had the opportunity to work with many challenges in this area. Over the years all of the physicians in what now has become NeuroCare Network, have entrusted us with many different types of spine patients. We have had the privilege to gain a tremendous experience base in spine care that we want to share with others. Because most all interventions for spine problems are controversial, there are often barriers in information exchange based on fear of criticism. We appreciate the efforts of many spine care professionals in East Texas who made sure that lines of communication remained open and active so we could work as a team.

We owe a great debt of gratitude to the physicians who have supported our therapy departments in this endeavor: Jonathan Blau, M.D., Aaron Calodney, M.D., Stuart Crutchfield, M.D., Guy Danielson, M.D., Ronald Donaldson, M.D., Paul Dreyfuss, M.D., Gary Eaton, D.O., Suzanne Fisher, M.D., David Fletcher, M.D., Charles Gordon, M.D., Jon Ledlie, M.D., James Michaels, M.D., Kevin Pauza, M.D., and Claire Tibiletti, M.D.

We also want to recognize the therapists who helped with the development and review of these protocols: Sheri Bjork, P.T., M.B.A., Carla Gleaton, M.Ed., P.T., Katy Hall, P.T., M.S., Carla Holmen, P.T.A., Clark Hopkins, P.T., Eddie Howard, P.T., M.B.A., Doug Jansen, D.P.T., Kevin Johns, P.T., M.S., Lee Johnson, P.T., Dennis Kress, P.T.A., Tom Lorren, P.T., Alejandro Ramirez, P.T., M.S., David Penn, P.T., O.C.S, Lee Spence, P.T., M.B.A., and Pam Thompson, P.T.

Joyce Ballard, Ph.D, exercise physiologist, played an important role in helping us with development of the cardiovascular testing and training sections. We would like to thank her for working with us.

In addition, we thank Shanda Troquille for patiently posing for all of our exercise photographs, many of which required several "takes."

We are grateful for the support from American Back Society throughout the protocol development process and especially for their sponsorship of this book. Our interaction with spine care professionals across the country began because of Aubrey Swartz, M.D., the Executive Director of American Back Society. He encouraged interaction and further study from the beginning of the work on the protocols. We especially appreciate Dr. Swartz for his support in the completion of this project. We also thank Dr. Philip E. Greenman for giving us the honor of reviewing our work and authoring our foreword.

Finally we would like to thank Michele Chase for her work of editing the book and for the ideas and support she gave throughout the process. We acknowledge the group at North Atlantic Books as well: Richard Grossinger, Susan Bumps, Brooke Warner, and Jan Camp, who were all very helpful in the production of the book, and wish to thank Nancy Humphreys and J. Naomi Linzer for indexing services.

Introduction

Why is rehabilitation important after spine surgery? Although most readers already know the answer, those who work with patients undergoing spine surgery are confronted with this question again and again. That the patient would need some rebuilding efforts after invading muscle, ligament, nerve, and often bone, not to mention after a significant period of pain-inhibited movement, would seem to go without saying. Unfortunately, in the case of many postsurgical spine patients, care is focused on crisis occurrences, and many times the care stops there.

Present day health care has been responsible for these trends, and physicians are necessarily focused on the most urgent needs with little time left for overall care. The allied health professionals may assume responsibility for these other levels of care, but they too must justify the time involved. So we find that the importance of rehabilitation must be reinforced with patients who may not appreciate benefits right away and physicians who are also concerned if benefits are not seen immediately. The difficulty of slow results with therapy, as compared to the immediate changes seen with medications and sometimes surgery, can discourage participants who do not fully understand the goal of rebuilding in rehabilitation. We also find ourselves defending therapies to insurance companies. Therapists are continuously challenged to their place in the front lines for these patients. (For more on these issues, see the appendix: "Rehabilitation of Patients Undergoing Spine Surgery in the Eyes of Physicians, Patients, and Payers: A Physical Therapy Challenge.")

Fortunately, the evidence in favor of spine rehabilitation is slowly building (Brennan et al. 1994; Hinkley and Jaremko 1997; Mayer et al. 1998; Nelson et al. 1999; O'Sullivan et al. 1997, Potvin and

O'Brien 1998; Richardson et al. 1999). On a daily basis, those of us in the clinic observe substantial benefits from rehabilitation in our patients following spine surgery. Over the years some of our local therapists have worked with hundreds and now thousands of post-surgical patients and have developed the protocols which form the basis of this book. We believe it may be unrealistic, however, to expect to be able to do controlled studies in our clinical settings. There is simply too much variability between day-to-day conditions for service delivery in a busy therapy department. Patients are often involved with more than one clinician as well as a variety of support staff members. However, one way busy clinics can contribute to research is by reporting clinical observations. We feel our accumulated information forms a strong base of ideas, tried but unproven, which we now want to share with other clinicians. We are hoping controlled studies might eventually be done where some of our ideas can be proven or discarded.

The initial work on these protocols began about eight years ago. Therapists working with competitive groups of surgeons decided to try and develop one program and maintain consistency on the rehabilitation level. Both groups of surgeons approved of the program we developed. Therapists throughout the region who cared for these surgeons' patients attended orientation sessions and workshops to learn the protocols. As we used this program and as surgeries changed, we modified the protocols. The principles behind the protocols remained basically the same, so we have tried to describe them in enough detail that they can be used simply by applying them. We have shared these protocols with therapists throughout our region, we now want to do this more formally and more widely.

Continuing challenges that will inevitably occur will include:
- spine surgeons forgetting to order rehabilitation for their patients;

- a feeling that surgery is the end of the line for some patients, and no other work should be done afterwards;

- a lack of appreciation for the increased complexity of a spine rehabilitation program which must necessarily consider neurologic as well as orthopedic concerns, more so perhaps, than other types of orthopedic patients (Richardson et al. 1999);

- some very complex mechanical problems as a result of years of chronic dysfunction, deconditioning, and then changes brought about by the surgery; and

- considerable difficulty in determining when rehabilitation is no longer justified. (We will give some tools to help with this determination in this book.)

Many times, therapists see postsurgical patients without knowing what surgery was done. Throughout this book, we strongly encourage therapists to find out as much detail as possible about the surgery. The operative report is very helpful, as it often describes the degree of difficulty, status of the involved tissues, and whether the patient had complications. All of these can help the therapist tailor the postsurgical program so the patient is not overloaded and the therapy unsuccessful from the start. Special attention can be given to selected tissues in the treatment program. Also, knowing the approach (location and size of incision), which muscles were invaded, the condition of the involved nerves, where bone grafts were obtained, and which type of hardware was used can all be used in making choices with rehabilitation. Our goal with this book is to make these considerations a routine part of decision making for the therapy program.

Abbreviations and Terms

Definitions are given in terms which are applicable to our protocols and in this book. These terms may be used differently in other contexts.

ABS   American Back Society

ACSM American College of Sports Medicine

ADL   activities of daily living

ALIF   anterior lumbar interbody fusion

APTA American Physical Therapy Association

BAK™ brand name of cage implant used for lumbar fusions. Some of our physicians were involved in the FDA studies for this in the mid 1990s.

DTR   deep tendon reflex

EDI   Electronic Digital Inclinometer (tm) (brand name of Cybex Company)

EMS   electrical muscle stimulation

ESI   epidural steroid injection

FCE   Functional Capacity Evaluation

Functional Loss Characteristics
    Described in Chapter 1: four categories of functional loss used to select spine stabilization exercise. Categories include: position sensitivity, pressure sensitivity, stasis sensitivity, and weight-bearing sensitivity.

HNP   herniated nucleus pulposus

IDET   Intradiscal Electrothermal Therapy

Inclinometer
A "bubble goniometer" device used for measuring spinal motion and postural curves

Kyphosis
On evaluation forms in this book, kyphosis refers to the inclinometer measure of the angle represented by the tangent lines to the ends of the thoracic curve, or from cervicothoracic junction to thoracolumbar junction.

LD (fascia)   lumbodorsal fascia

Lordosis
On evaluation forms in this book, lordosis refers to the inclinometer measure of the angle represented by the tangent lines to the ends of the lumbar curve, or from thoracolumbar junction to lumbosacral junction.

MET   metabolic equivalent (oxygen consumption required): a unit of measurement of energy requirement for a given activity, expressed as a MET level.

MMI   maximum medical improvement

MMPI   Minnesota Multiphasic Personality Inventory

PCT   Physical Capacities Test

PEP   Presurgical Evaluation Program

PLF   posterior lateral fusion

PLIF   posterior lumbar interbody fusion

PSIS posterior superior iliac spine

SLR straight leg raise

Segmental stabilization

> Refers to exercise designed to condition muscles which can offer support and control of movement on a vertebra-by-vertebra basis in the spine. This term has been studied and defined more elaborately in a text on this subject released recently (Richardson et al. 1999).

Spine stabilization

> Refers to exercise (referenced in Chapters 1 and 10), designed to create a muscular system of optimal support for the spine which can offer protection during maintained positions or movement.

TENS transcutaneous electrical nerve stimulation

TLSO thoraco-lumbo-sacral orthosis

ULTT upper limb tension test

Work hardening:

> A program used to physically prepare for return to work by simulating job duties and having the individual perform the duties on a repeated basis for reconditioning. Most work hardening programs also prepare the patient for return to an eight hour work day by attending the program on a full time basis.

Chapter One

•••••••••••••••

Nonsurgical and Presurgical Management of Patients with Spine Pathologies

APPROACHES TO WORK WITH LUMBAR SPINE PATHOLOGIES

A great deal has been written on the subject of nonsurgical spine treatment, and several references are included on this subject in the annotated bibliography at the end of the book. In this chapter, a general protocol for initial management of the spine patient will be outlined. Our purpose in beginning with a nonsurgical protocol is to introduce our general approach to working with lumbar spine pathologies. Our approach is an eclectic one which can accommodate differing schools of thought about methods or practice. The ideas in these protocols are presented in an attempt to develop common time frames, parameters for progress, and indications for referral to another practitioner. Also, we attempted to leave room for those therapists in multidisciplinary practices who may be sharing the care of the patient with other disciplines.

Our group of therapists found the most universal language for describing the spine patient's symptoms in the *functional loss characteristics* defined in the first spine stabilization programs, specifically in one from the San Francisco Spine Institute (Robinson 1991; Saal 1991). Almost any decrease in function, secondary to spinal pain or dysfunction, can be described in terms of the four characteristics listed in Figure 1. There we have described functional losses, with examples of ways to overcome them in the treatment program. The goal of the therapist is almost always to design the program around eliminating each loss (Biondi 1991; Morgan 1988).

Figure 1. Functional Loss Characteristics and Associated Activity Modifications

I. Weight-bearing sensitivity: The patient has most pain in upright, especially with standing and walking. Sometimes it is unilateral with leg pain; sometimes bilateral with back, buttock, or hip pain. *Strategies:*
   A. Start with non-weight-bearing exercise, sitting, lying down, or in a pool.
   B. Allow for frequent position changes when upright.
   C. Strictly enforce lifting limit, as lifting adds to the weight-bearing load.
   D. Measure progress with walking distance possible without leg pain or other significant weight-bearing pain.

II. Position sensitivity: Pain occurs when spine is either flexed, extended, or laterally flexed. This is also described by McKenzie (1991) as *directional preference*. In the case of position sensitivity, the position *to be avoided* is described. *Strategies:*

A. Select spine stabilization exercises with flexion bias for extension sensitivity, and vice versa. For patients with sensitivity to both flexion and extension, stabilization should be done close to neutral position.

B. Use mobilization to facilitate return of sensitive motions, but be sure that peripheral symptoms do not occur.

C. Reinforce lifting limit. Limit compression forces to the spine which may increase a position sensitivity.

D. Try backward walking or cycling with the extension sensitive patient. Often patients with spinal stenosis will be extension sensitive.

III. Pressure sensitivity: Pain occurs with surface pressure and often is due to soft tissue involvement. *Strategies:*

A. Use ice, ultrasound, or electrical stimulation to decrease the sensitivity.

B. Modify exercises to avoid additional pressure on the area: i.e. abdominal work is often painful for patients with pressure sensitivity over the spinous processes if the low back is not on a cushioned surface.

C. Encourage aerobic work to help overall oxygenation of tissues, increase blood flow to accelerate healing and diminish pain from ischemia.

IV. Stasis sensitivity: Sensitivity occurs with maintained positions. *Strategies:*

A. This is the best advertisement for exercise and therapy, so recommend them!

B. Educate the patient regarding oscillatory motions and benefits from small repeated motions decreasing overall forces on joints.

C. Use spine stabilization incorporating as much mobility as possible.

Our techniques and philosophies throughout this book incorporate many concepts presented by Robin McKenzie, O.B.E., F.N.Z. (1991) and also by Stanley Paris, Ph.D., P.T. (1985, 1998), keeping in mind that these individuals have fairly divergent viewpoints at times. They have both made major contributions in improving therapists' evaluation skills and treatment options for spinal problems, and that knowledge supports clinicians' effectiveness. Our program probably most closely parallels the approach of Saunders (1994) or a more traditional orthopedic therapy practice (Basmajian and Nyberg 1993; Greenman 1996).

The "Acute Protocol" shown in Figure 2 lists many alternatives for treatment choices in the various stages of patient care. The protocol assumes the treatment plan corresponds to the evaluation findings, as described in Chapter 2.

Figure 3 gives an example of a progress note which we designed for manual therapists to indicate their emphasis on a particular visit. There are three columns with Roman numerals found in the middle section of the form to describe manual work in up to three different areas, for example, lumbar spine, pelvis, and lower extremity. Below these sections the therapist might indicate which techniques were used, such as Grade II PA pressures, pelvic muscle energy techniques, and neural mobilization, respectively. The patients' responses to treatment can be documented in the "comments" section. The form also has space to document patient education, a key part of the program. The exercise portion of the note is a summary of what is actually recorded in detail, on a flow sheet in our case. There is space following the exercise checklist to add comments about patient responses also. In Chapter 10 of this book, sample flow sheets and exercise routine examples are included.

Please pay particular attention to section III of the protocol outline. This section lists signs and symptoms which should indicate referral back to the physician. These may vary significantly between physicians, and therefore must be verified with referring physicians in each case. Be ready to discover some vague information in this area. If therapists are unable to pin physicians down on definite red flags, they should make their own list and have them agree or disagree. This is how we finally arrived at our list. There is no doubt in our experience that having a red flag list of some sort can be a great safety feature for a program.

It is important to note in all protocols that much of the treatment selection is based on evaluation findings. We cover presurgical evaluation in the next section and postsurgical evaluation in the next chapter, and much of this can be applied to the nonsurgical patient as well. Once again, depending on the therapist's background with spine care, other methods of evaluation can be used and adapted to these protocols.

Figure 2: Protocol for Nonsurgical and Presurgical Spine Management

I. **Rehabilitation Goals,** weeks 1-6 following evaluation.
  A. Minimize symptoms and progression of pathology.
  B. Assess capacity for activities of daily living (ADLs) and work.
  C. Promote soft tissue and structural healing.
  D. Initiate activity-based management.

II. **Rehabilitation Program,** weeks 1-6.
  A. Carry out evaluation, including assessment of functional loss characteristics.
  B. Control symptoms.

1. Position, protect, and support
2. Make use of appropriate modalities as needed for pain control. Decrease usage as function improves.
3. Begin back education process, and document topics discussed with the patient in daily notes.
4. Limit lifting to ten pounds until patient is able to pass Level I spine stabilization screens (not done until pain is controlled).
5. Introduce temporary bracing if support helps with pain control (which also may facilitate restoration of activity).
6. Utilize a TENS unit, or portable EMS, emphasizing temporary usage for pain control, if it enables the patient to function with less medication.
7. Coordinate care with chiropractor, when applicable. Avoid duplication of modalities. Communicate therapy and chiropractic goals to be sure they work together for the patient.

C. Start corrective exercises once symptoms are controlled.

1. Spine stabilization exercises selected with consideration of functional loss characteristics. Begin with Level I, fully supported, then progress to less supported.
2. Aerobic training, starting with walking, unless patient is weight- bearing sensitive, in which case, try either cycling (especially recumbent cycling) or pool walking.
3. Corrective stretching, including neural mobilization.
4. Functional activity practice using proper body mechanics, with repetition to help habit change. See functional activity sheet (Figure 33) in Chapter 10.

III. *RE-EVALUATE AND RETURN TO DOCTOR AT ANY POINT IF:*

A. Neurologic signs are increased for forty-eight hours or more. These may include deep tendon reflex change, significant change in nerve tension tests, strength loss in a muscle group, or sensory change.

B. Neurologic signs show any indications of cord compression or other upper motor neuron sign, such as:

1. Lhermitte's sign;

2. new Babinski or clonus noted;

3. changes in bowel, bladder, or sexual function;

4. sudden diffuse motor loss;

5. other signs as indicated by surgeon involved. Different surgeons have different areas of concern and tests of importance.

C. No progress in any PCT category (see Chapter 3) at two weeks, or four weeks in categories where some changes would be expected.

D. Patient shows indications of psychological overlay during the first two weeks of therapy. The physician should be alerted at this point and may not require an appointed visit.

IV. **Rehabilitation Goals,** week six until therapy discharge.

A. Assign advanced exercise to prepare for return to work and activity prior to injury.

B. Continue to reinforce proper body mechanics and back maintenance as habit.

C. Try to establish ongoing exercise as lifelong habit.

D. Reach point of Maximum Medical Improvement (MMI) in the shortest feasible time frame, especially if patient is on workers' compensation.

V. **Rehabilitation Program,** week six until therapy discharge.

A. Continue progression of all types of exercise described in section II with Physical Capacities Tests every two weeks to quantify progress. (See next chapter.)

B. Continue back education, and document topics each visit.

C. Continue to reinforce the benefits of exercise to the patient.

D. Carry out Functional Capacity Evaluation and follow-up on areas failed or return to work and discharge.

PRESURGICAL EVALUATION PROGRAM (PEP)

PEP was designed and implemented in response to the growing awareness within the medical community of the complexities involved in successful surgical treatment of the patient with spine injury. It has become apparent to the surgical specialist that successful intervention requires a more comprehensive approach that is sensitive to the human impact issues as well as the physical issues. The current program attempts to discern those issues that predictably impact both surgical appropriateness and outcome.

The presurgical evaluation program serves three functions:

1. to educate patients about spine care and pre- and post-operative issues;

2. to rate patients according to the probability of successful surgical outcome based upon anatomical defect severity, potential for surgical success in correcting the patient's anatomical defect, and psychosocial factors (rated by both psychologist and physical therapist); and

3. to make recommendations to the spine injured patient concerning the most appropriate route of managing spine-related pain.

Figure 4 outlines a schedule of evaluations, as we do it at the East Texas Medical Center.

NeuroCare Network
PHYSICAL MEDICINE DEPARTMENT
816 S. Fleishel
Tyler, Texas 75701
(903)597-3472

Therapist's Notes

Visit #:_____

Patient:_____ Date:_____

S: _____
_____
_____
_____

O: Exercises performed (see flow sheet for details):   Time:_____
Area as described in PLAN OF CARE: ☐ Stretching   ☐ Aerobic Training   ☐ Other: _____
                                     ☐ Strength   ☐ Balance and Coordination   ☐ Spine Stabilization   _____
Modifications to Program (PROGRESSION): _____
_____

ONE-TO-ONE MANUAL THERAPY WITH THE THERAPIST/PTA AS FOLLOWS:
                    I   II   III
Area:_____
Type:_____
_____
_____
_____

Goal:_____
_____

Comment:_____
_____

Measurement/Tests: _____
_____

Patient Education: _____
_____

MODALITIES:
Electrical Stim:_____   Ultrasound:_____   Other: _____
Parameters/Intensity: _____
Purpose: ☐ for Pain Control   ☐ Muscle Facilitation   ☐ Tissue Healing
                ☐ To Increase Circulation   ☐ Swelling
                ☐ Other:_____
A: Goals addressed today:_____
_____

Remaining Deficits: _____
P: _____
_____
_____
_____

_____
Therapist

Figure 3:Sample Progress Note Form

Figure 4: PEP Schedule

A. Day 1 (8:00 A.M. until testing completed)
   1. Psychological testing
   2. Physical therapy evaluation
   3. Psychologist's personal interview

B. Day 2 - Educational sessions (8:00 A.M.- 3:00 P.M.)
   1. Pain medications: 30 min. (registered nurse)
   2. Anatomy of spine, disc pathology, and basic explanation of spine surgeries: 2 hrs. 30 min. (physical therapist)
   3. Psychological issues which can affect surgical outcome: 1 hr. (psychologist)
   4. One hour lunch for patients; physical therapist and psychologist meet to discuss findings.
   5. Factors that contribute to spine related pain: 2 hrs. (physical therapist)

C. Day 3 (6:30 A.M. until staffing completed)
   1. 6:30 A.M. Conference with physicians and PEP team presenting detail of each participating patient. Patients each accepted or not accepted as surgical candidate. Follow-up recommendations made.
   2. Individual conference with each patient is done and psychologist discusses recommendations.

PSYCHOLOGICAL TESTING AND INTERVIEW

Three types of psychological testing are used in our program. These are fairly commonly known and widely used tests, including Minnesota Multiphasic Personality Inventory (MMPI), Wahler Physical Symptoms Inventory, and Personal Problems Checklist. These tests are used to determine the patient's personality profile and can help guide the physician's surgical or nonsurgical recommendations.

A personal interview with each patient is also performed by the psychologist. This interview includes but is not limited to the following aspects of the patient history: medical, educational, marital, legal, and pharmaceutical.

PHYSICAL THERAPY EVALUATION

A physical therapist evaluates each patient in the PEP program. There are two goals of this evaluation: to check the patient's general physical state and to observe any exaggeration of symptoms. A preprinted form entitled *PEP Lumbar Assessment* is shown in Figure 5 and is meant to be a guide for the evaluation. This evaluation is typically not as extensive as one we might perform in an outpatient clinic setting since the goals are somewhat different. During the evaluation a brief video is made of each patient performing simple lumbar and lower extremity exercises. The patient's capability to move between various sitting and recumbent positions can be observed. Gait is filmed as well.

PHYSICAL THERAPY PRESURGICAL RATING GUIDE

For several years an attempt to explain the physical therapy rating score to the physicians without a guide met with mixed success. A few years ago, the guide found in Figure 6 was developed, and the physicians seemed to accept this system more readily. The following is a brief description of each item on the guide.

1. OVERWEIGHT

Although it has not been proven that being overweight is a direct contributing factor to back problems, it may speak to the patient's

LUMBAR ASSESSMENT

NAME_____ AGE_____ HT_____ WT_____

BP_____ DATE OF INJURY_____ SMOKE? (AMT)_____

EMPLOYER AT DOI_____ HOW LONG EMPLOYED PTI?_____

JOB DESCRIPTION (TITLE)_____

DESCRIPTION OF INJURY_____

BACK/NECK SURGERIES (& DATES)_____

PREVIOUS P.T.? (PLACE)_____

LEVEL OF EDUCATION_____

AMBITIONS: PLAN ON RETURNING TO PREVIOUS JOB?_____
                      IF NOT, PLANS?_____

PAIN COMPLAINTS: RATING_____ % SPINE/EXTR'S_____

POSTURE: KYPH_____ LORD_____

ROM: FLEX_____ EXT_____ SBR_____ SBL_____

STRENGTH: GRIP: RIGHT_____ LEFT_____
                      REG INCREASED?_____ RIGHT_____ LEFT_____

                LE"S: HIP FLEX   QUADS   ANKLE DF   EHL   GASTROC
                      RT   _____   _____   _____   _____   _____
                      LT   _____   _____   _____   _____   _____

                HEEL WALK:_____ TOE WALK:_____ (YES OR NO)

GAIT (COMMENTS)_____

SLR: R_____ PAIN LOC._____ L_____ PAIN LOC_____

WADDELL SIGNS: PALPATION_____ NON-ANAT_____
                DISTRACT_____ SIMULATION_____ OVERREACT_____

OVERLY DRAMATIC VERBAL AND PHYSICAL PAIN BEHAVIOR?_____

Figure 5. PEP Lumbar Assessment Form

self-discipline and general physical condition. It is believed that a significant number of patients could decrease their back pain if they lost weight and started a regular exercise program.

The last one hundred males evaluated in our program averaged forty-one pounds overweight using the Metropolitan Life Insurance Company adult height and weight charts. The females averaged thirty-three pounds overweight.

The rating guide assigns a number of *risk* points that increases with amount overweight.

2. BLOOD PRESSURE

This factor reflects general physical condition, but if elevated, can present a potential factor which can represent surgical risk as well as a potential slowed recovery. If the patient's diastolic pressure is above one hundred, it can be indicative of uncontrolled blood pressure whether or not the patient is taking medication for the problem. Blood pressure problems often limit the rate of progression with exercise and reconditioning. Risk points are assigned as shown in the guide form for high blood pressure.

3. SMOKING

Smoking has been associated with higher risk for back pain in general, poor outcome with back surgery, and specifically to the likelihood of nonfusion (Silcox et al. 1995). Smoking cessation is therefore heavily stressed during the presurgical education sessions. It is recommended that patients should stop smoking for at least three months following the surgery. Points are assigned for the amount the patient admits to smoking, as our experience is that patients who smoke more are less likely to try to stop.

4. LENGTH OF TIME OFF WORK

There are many statistics available that indicate pessimistic outlooks for those individuals who have been off work for six months or more (Skinner 1993). Percentages decline even more for those who are off one to two years (Blankenship 1990). Unfortunately, surgery for individuals without a future occupation can represent another reason not to ever try to return to work.

5. ATTORNEY INVOLVEMENT WITH THE BACK INJURY CLAIM

Legal entanglement may affect surgical outcome by increasing the patient's stress level and by secondary gain issues. Attorney involvement is therefore considered a risk factor. The psychologist assesses the patient in this area and can be of assistance with this rating.

6. GAIT EXHIBITING SYMPTOM MAGNIFICATION

Gait with gross abnormalities, sometimes requiring more effort than normal gait, can represent a *red flag*. Gait on the video can be observed for consistency in other situations. This is a subjective rating on the part of the therapist. Points are assigned to the patient if symptom magnification is observed during gait, or if inconsistent gait patterns are observed. We have noticed that the surgeons appreciate the video for this purpose and often will judge the video on their own.

7. PAIN DRAWING

The pain drawing can also indicate signs of symptom magnification. Various methods of rating pain drawings are presented by different authors (Rothman and Simeone 1992). The one used in our rating guide is from Blankenship (1990).Generally, too much detail on the pain drawing can indicate symptom magnification.

8. WADDELL SIGNS

These nonorganic physical signs were originally described by Waddell et al. in 1980, and have an established history in the spine field. The *Waddell Signs* are widely utilized and known by many spine specialists. According to Waddell, if three or more of the five signs are positive, the patient may benefit from psychological intervention. More recently, these signs have been considered by some to be controversial due to potential variability in testing and interpretation (Lechner et al. 1998). In our rating scale, we have found them helpful, so we assign risk points to those patients with three or more positive Waddell Signs.

9. STRAIGHT LEG RAISE TEST POSITIVE BELOW TWENTY DEGREES.

The straight leg test description from the 1800s has been studied further in current spine texts (Borenstein and Weisel 1989). The opinion is that the pain arises when an irritated sciatic nerve is stretched as the leg is raised from the supine position. It is believed that the nerve does not stretch until the leg is raised above an angle of thirty to thirty-five degrees (of hip flexion with knee extended). According to Borenstein and Weisel the stretch occurs from about thirty to seventy degrees.

A patient who reports pain out of the range of stretch on the nerve is considered a possible symptom magnifier.

10. BACK TO WORK ISSUES

A major purpose of many spine surgeries is to return a person to employment. A person may not be able to return to their previous occupation; however, the verbalization of a plan to return to work is considered a positive sign. Likewise, the lack of a plan is considered another risk for poorer outcome.

PHYSICAL THERAPY PEP RATING GUIDE

1. OVERWEIGHT
   10-29 LBS.......... 2
   30-49 LBS.......... 5
   50-69 LBS.......... 9
   70-89 LBS.......... 14
   >89 LBS.......... 20

2. BLOOD PRESSURE
   DIASTOLIC>100..... 5

3. SMOKING
   <.5 PACK/DAY................. 5
   .5 - 1.5 PACK/DAY........... 10
   >1.5 PACK/DAY............... 20

4. HOW LONG OFF WORK?
   STILL WORKING OR
   OFF WORK <6 MOS........ 0
   6MOS - 1 YR..................... 5
   >1 YR............................... 10
   >2 YR............................... 20

5. DOES PATIENT HAVE AN
   ATTORNEY INVOLVED IN
   THEIR BACK INJURY
   CLAIM?
   APPEARS TO BE OF:
   MINIMAL CONCERN........ 0
   MOD TO MAX
   INVOLVMENT................... 10

6. GAIT APPEARS TO EXHIBIT
   MAGNIFIED PAIN BEHAVIOR.
   MINIMAL............................. 5
   OVERT............................... 10

7. PAIN DRAWING:
   SCORED ACCORDING TO
   BLANKENSHIP'S INSTRUCTIONS
   THREE................................ 5
   FOUR.................................. 10
   FIVE OR MORE.................. 15

8. WADDELL SIGNS:
   ONE POSITIVE.................... 0
   TWO POSITIVE................... 0
   THREE POSITIVE................ 5
   FOUR POSITIVE.................. 9
   FIVE POSITIVE.................... 14

9. SLR TEST POSITIVE BELOW 20 .. 10

10. BACK TO WORK ISSUES:
    HAS JOB TO RETURN TO AND
    PLANNING TO RETURN.............. 0
    NO JOB TO RETURN TO BUT
    HAS PLANS FOR EMPLOYMENT
    AND/OR HAS CONTACTED TRC...* 5
    VAGUE, UNREALISTIC PLANS
    FOR EMPLOYMENT......................... 10
    NO GOALS FOR EMPLOYMENT
    AND/OR HAS APPLIED FOR
    SS DISABILITY................................... 15

   0 -- 4 POINTS..........EXCELLENT............ 5
   5 -- 14 POINTS.......GOOD....................... 4
   15 -- 24 POINTS........FAIR........................ 3
   25 -- 50 POINTS.........POOR....................... 2
   >50 POINTS.................VERY POOR............ 1

*TRC—Texas Rehabilitation Commission

Figure 6. Physical Therapy PEP Rating Guide

RATING USING THE PHYSICAL THERAPY GUIDE

A rating of 5 or *excellent* tells the physician that the patient appears to be in good general condition and there is no noticeable symptom magnification or potential psychological barrier to recovery from surgery. A rating of 4 or *good* describes a patient in good or fair general condition with little or no symptom magnification. There may be a specific area of concern that needs to be addressed after surgery. A rating of 3 or *fair* describes a patient who exhibits several areas of risk with regard to physical condition and/or symptom magnification. These areas of risk usually need to be addressed either before or after the surgery to maximize the surgical benefit. A rating of 2 or 1, *poor* or *very poor* respectively, describes a patient who probably has significant physical and psychological risk factors. Patients with these lower ratings are often referred for physical conditioning and/or psychological counseling prior to surgery.

The physical therapy rating is utilized as a guide and is not a definitive parameter for exclusion or clearance for spine surgery. There is a large component of judgment by the therapist based on the testing and the patient's cooperation and interest in the educational component of the program.

CONFERENCE WITH THE PHYSICIANS AND PEP TEAM

In an average one and one-half hour PEP staffing meeting there are usually eight to ten physicians present. These may include neurosurgeons, orthopedic surgeons, nonsurgical spine specialists, and one radiologist. The PEP team consists of a nurse, psychologist, and physical therapist who have interacted with the patients. Visitors to the staffing may include case managers, physician's office nurses, and visiting physicians. Due to patient confidentiality issues, other visitors are not allowed in the staffing. Staffings begin with a patient's prospective surgeon presenting a brief history of the case.

The radiologist then shows what he or she considers relevant radiology scans with an overhead projector on a large screen at the front of the room. After physician discussion, the prospective surgeon rates the anatomical defect and the potential for surgical success in correcting the anatomical defect using the scales found in Figure 7. The physical therapist then presents a brief summary of his or her evaluation and gives the physical therapy rating previously described. The therapist also shows the video of the patient taken during the evaluation. The psychologist then gives a brief summary of findings from the psychological testing and interview. The psychological rating is also from 1 to 5, with 1 as poor and 5 as excellent.

SUMMARY OF THE PEP PROGRAM

The PEP program has been a useful screening system for patients who are candidates for lumbar spine surgery. It can help identify areas of risk before the surgery, and lessen chances of complications or poor outcome. The system has yet to be fully proven, and therefore may be denied payment by some insurance plans. However, given the current general frequency of suboptimal surgical outcome, presurgical screening is an important area for further research.

PEP RATING SCALE

#1. ANATOMICAL DEFECT SEVERITY SCALE

1. QUESTIONABLE OR NO PATHOLOGY

2. MINIMAL PATHOLOGY-e.g.   DISC BULGE

3. MODERATE PATHOLOGY-e.g.   HNP
SINGLE LEVEL DDD
GRADE I SPONDYLOLISTHESIS

4. SIGNIFICANT PATHOLOGY-e.g. HNP
TWO LEVEL DDD
GRADE II SPONDYLOLISTHESIS

5. EXTREME PATHOLOGY-e.g.   HNP
MULTIPLE LEVEL DDD
> GRADE II SPONDYLOLISTHESIS

#2. FOR SPINE SURGERY PATIENTS-POTENTIAL FOR SURGICAL SUCCESS IN CORRECTING THE PATIENT'S ANATOMICAL DEFECT

1. POOR

2. FAIR

3. MODERATE

4. SIGNIFICANT

5. EXCELLENT

Figure 7. PEP Rating Scales

Chapter Two

•··•❶•••••••••

Evaluating the Patient
Following Lumbar Spine Surgery

Evaluation of the postsurgical patient is often complicated by the great variation in time frame between surgery and initial therapy order. History-taking is a key component, as always, and is most helpful if it differentiates current symptoms from those which were present presurgically. A much larger range of "normal" symptoms follows surgery and may last for several weeks, creating more difficulty in deciding what conditions require earlier referral back to the surgeon. History-taking for spine patients has been well described by several authors (Basmajian and Nyberg 1993; Corrigan and Maitland 1985; Magee 1987; McKenzie 1991; Richardson and Iglarsh 1994). Almost every text on spine treatment has complete information on history-taking so it will not be covered in depth here.

There are some important history items to include postsurgically:

1. nature, distribution, and duration of the pain currently; nature of the pain refers to type of pain(s), frequency, intensity, and duration of pain episodes;

2. nature, distribution and duration of the pain before surgery;

3. positions or conditions which improve or worsen the pain;

4. presence of bowel or bladder symptoms, or other systemic complaints;

5. comorbidities which may affect exercise selection, and

6. activities which are currently limited, which were not limited before the symptom onset, and also since surgery. This can serve as a check of the patient's understanding of their postoperative restrictions as well.

The physical therapy evaluation follows and is designed to make a physical therapy diagnosis which can be well described in terms of the functional loss characteristics covered in the previous chapter. A specific therapeutic program based on the patient's individual needs can then be made and combined with forces which can help the healing surgery. Adjustments to the program can be made based on the patient's responses to treatment and be recorded to describe progression. In this way the physical therapist functions to provide ongoing differential diagnosis information for the surgeon as well as to assure the best rehabilitation path for the patient.

A copy of our current evaluation form is found in Figure 8. Evolution of evaluation forms is an ongoing process, especially as there is more communication between clinicians regarding rehabilitation following spine surgeries. Brief descriptions of methods involved in the evaluation follow. (Some methods are described in detail elsewhere in the book.) We have selected a narrow range from many existing evaluation techniques to work toward consistency in our reporting, but this does not mean other evaluation techniques cannot work just as well. Most evaluation tools have limitations. Discussion of one widely used measurement tool, inclinometer measurement, is included at the end of this chapter for consideration. We believe that description of motion in the spine is key to a complete evaluation, and we advocate any attempt to improve upon use of spine measurement tools for clinical meaningfulness.

LUMBAR POSTSURGICAL EVALUATION FORM

In the first section, a few patient demographics are needed. The type and date of surgery should include as much information as possible, including spinal levels operated on, fusion or nonfusion, anterior or posterior approach, and with or without hardware (for fusion surgeries). Again, attaching the surgical report to this form is the best case scenario. Pain medication lists can be helpful information and sometimes can account for unexpected responses to treatment.

At this point, note the check-boxes along the left hand margin of the evaluation form. These are to be checked if an abnormality is found in the corresponding section of the evaluation. The check-boxes can be used to be certain all evaluation findings are addressed in the plan of care.

There is a space on the form for gait description, and it is helpful at this point to document any use of a cane or walker. Gait can simply be checked as *normal* or checked if deviations are noted. It is helpful to give a short description such as *antalgic* or *ataxic,* or *further analysis recommended.*

Grip strength is measured with a grip dynamometer and is a measurement used to monitor consistency and level of effort. We recommend checking grip strength on every visit as a means of monitoring consistency. Use the left hand check-box if the grip strength shows significant asymmetry or abnormally low values.

Posture measurement and documentation techniques are covered in the inclinometer portion of this chapter. Active lumbar range of motion is covered in this section also. Please refer to this section for details.

Spine inspection includes a careful documentation of the status of the incision site and the soft tissue of the lumbar spine area. The incision location, size, and orientation on the body can be helpful. With anterior approach surgeries, vertical incision versus anterior oblique incision changes the muscles invaded. There are also spaces to describe discoloration, drainage (amount, color, and odor) and skin temperature. *Lumbar spine contour* should include descriptions of any soft tissue masses, horizontal tissue bands across the spine, or steps noted when palpating the spinous processes. Paraspinal muscle performance *refers to palpation of active contraction with comparison between right and left sides. This may or may not be possible to assess at the postoperative evaluation, if the patient is having much discomfort. Indicate* test deferred due to pain *so it is clear the test was not simply omitted.*

Pertinent lower extremity range limitations should include a list of any significant right/left difference found at hip, knee, or ankle. Tight muscle groups in the extremities can be noted here as well. Foot pulses can help identify circulatory complications. The neurologic screen tests are described in the section on Physical Capacities testing, in Chapter 3.

USING INCLINOMETER MEASURES TO HELP DESCRIBE FUNCTION AND PROGRESS IN THE SPINE PATIENT

Inclinometer measures are described in the *AMA Guides to Evaluation of Permanent Impairment, Third Edition* (1988) and continue to be used for impairment assessments. Inclinometers are frequently found in clinics now and are probably the most commonly used measurement tool for assessing spinal mobility. Some companies have produced digital inclinometers, such as the Cybex EDI (tm), and some companies have computer software that will include some of the impairment calculations along with the motion

LUMBAR POSTSURGICAL EVALUATION Form

Patient name_____DOB_____Date_____

Date of procedure_____SURGERY (levels & type) _____

CHECK ONE: Pre-eval_____6 wk post_____other_____

PainMedications: (dose/how many per day?)

□ Gait: _____normal _____Deviation:_____

□ Grip Strength   R_____   L_____

□ Posture:_____kyphosis (norm, xs) _____lordosis (norm, xs) ; _____R / L lat shift

Asymm L/R: Head_____; shoulders_____; iliac_____; PSIS_____;legs/feet_____

Sagittal deviations: head_____; shoulders_____; trunk_____; pelvis_____;

□ **Spine Inspection:**   skin surface (scar description & location)_____

discoloration_____; drainage_____: temp_____

Lumbar spine contour (i.e. steps, soft tissue)_____

□ Paraspinal muscle performance_____

□ Active lumbar spinal motion:

Inclinometer ROM	ROM deviations/limitations	Pain Production
Flexion_____	_____	_____
Extension_____	_____	_____
Right lat _____	_____	_____
Left lat _____	_____	_____

□ Pertinent Lower Extremity ROM limitations:

□ Foot Pulses:_____

Neuro Screen

□   DTR's_____

□   SLR_____Femoral Nv._____

□   SENSORY_____

□   MOTOR_____

□   FUNCTIONAL MOBILITY: supine/sit/supine_____single leg balance_____

body mech pick-up_____; heel walk_____; toe walk_____; squat_____

□   Babinski _____; Clonus _____; other_____

□   **Functional Loss Characteristics:** weight bearing sensitivity_____; stasis sensitivity_____;

pressure sensitivity (location)_____; position sensitivity (direction)_____

Changes from previous evaluation:

PLAN: (include each checked item):

_____therapist _____dictated

Figure 8. Lumbar Postsurgical Evaluation Form

measures. Also, there are devices that will attach the inclinometer to an area for easier measure, such as the CROM (tm) and the BROM (tm). The CROM measures neck motion with the device strapped to the head, and the BROM measures back motion with the device strapped to the back. The principle of all of these devices is the same: the inclinometer takes angular measurements from a reference line, usually the line of gravity.

Lumbar lordosis can be measured by placing the inclinometer at the thoraco-lumbar (T-L) junction and at the sacrum and subtracting the difference in angles measured. The measurement at each of the sites is an angular measurement from the vertical reference. The inclinometers do have a movable scale so they can be "zeroed" at the first point and simply read at the second point to give the difference in angle between the two points. The angular measure between the two tangents at each end of the curve represents the measurement of the curve. In the thoracic spine, the thoracic kyphosis may be measured in a similar way by taking the tangent to the cervical-thoracic (C-T) junction and the T-L junction.

The AMA *Guides* (1988) recommend using two inclinometers, one at each end point of the region of interest, to minimize error from placing and replacing the inclinometers. The *Guides* describe motion measurement by placing the inclinometers at the two ends of the curve and "zeroing" both while the patient stands in a neutral posture. Readings are taken from each inclinometer when the patient bends as far forward as possible. Subtracting the sacral reading from the T-L junction reading is used to represent *true lumbar flexion:* the amount of flexion that occurs in the lumbar spine only, and not including motion at the hips or pelvis. Flexion is considered normal in impairment rating terms at sixty degrees. However, this amount of motion includes the patient moving out of their lordotic curve as part of the lumbar flexion measure. The lumbar spine may not appear to be bending forward much to have "normal" flexion, if there is much lordosis present.

Lumbar extension and lateral bending are measured with a similar method of zeroing the two inclinometers at T-L junction and sacrum, then subtracting the lower inclinometer reading from the upper to arrive at the measured amount. The method is similar with the thoracic spine. In the cervical spine, the upper cervical inclinometer is placed on the head so the measure becomes more indirect.

A disadvantage to the use of inclinometer measures is that the angular value is limited in describing a curved surface. Many times, especially with spine pathologies, the curved surface is irregular and, in fact, may show a significant abnormality in spite of a measure that falls within normal range. However, using added descriptors may be a way practitioners could continue to use this simple and easy measurement technique (moving toward more universal practice) and still make the measurements meaningful in the care path of the patient.

Below are some examples of both posture and motion abnormalities that could be clarified with descriptors. The motion or posture is quantified using the inclinometer measure, then qualified with the descriptor.

Postural Abnormality	Descriptor
thoracic irregularities	Flattened mid-thoracic spine
	Evidence of scoliosis or asymmetry
	Curvature concentrated at caudal or cephalad end of curve, or Dowager's hump included in measurement

lumbar irregularities   Sharp lumbosacral angle

Step or prominent vertebra

Previous surgical changes

Pelvic asymmetries

Irregular soft tissue, tissue band

Motion abnormalities in either the thoracic or lumbar spine may include rotation occurring in another plane during the measured movement (other than coupled movement), uneven motion distribution suggesting either restricted or unstable levels, and relative contribution of movement in the measured area to the overall movement (the lumbar or the thoracic spine may be the primary area bending in the measured direction). All of these factors can influence diagnosis and maximize mechanical management of the patient. Another very important descriptor is that of symptoms that occur with each movement. In order to include the information in a summarized form on evaluation, a recording sheet can be used as shown below. (Note: This recording form is part of the Lumbar Postsurgical Evaluation Form found in Figure 8)

Active Lumbar Range of Motion

	Inclin. ROM	ROM deviations/limitations	Pain production
Flexion	_____	_____	_____
Extension	_____	_____	_____
Right lat.	_____	_____	_____
Left lat.	_____	_____	_____

Some examples of lumbar spine measurement descriptors could include:

Flexion: "forty degrees . . . prominent lower lumbar vertebra noted . . . buttock and posterior thigh pain to knee." Of course, abbreviations can make this easy to record quickly. The prominent lower vertebra could alert the practitioner to a possible instability, or postsurgical change. The leg pain can help with differential diagnosis and can be used as a parameter for progress.

Flexion: "sixty degrees . . . forward bending limited fifty percent overall . . . mid-back pain noted." This patient is moving mostly in the lumbar spine, and is either restricted at the hips or the thoracic spine or both. This information may help with diagnosis and treatment selection.

Extension: "twenty-five degrees . . . some right rotation noted in the lower T-spine . . . right buttock pain." These descriptors could suggest some mechanical pain generators.

Chapter Three

•··•●●•••••••••

Interim Testing of the Spine Patient: The Physical Capacities Test

The Physical Capacities Test (PCT) was designed by our group of therapists to establish a uniform way of reporting progress on spine patients. We wanted to be able to briefly measure several parameters of progress weekly or every two weeks and show progress toward short term goals. The PCT form (Figure 9) was arranged in a chart form with columns for each test so that progress could be compared from week to week or from test to test. The test was designed to be used for either cervical or lumbar spine problems, and both will be described in this chapter. It was intended to be as simple as possible so that a physician could read it rapidly and see the areas where the patient was or was not progressing.

There are six main categories of tests on the PCT form:

1. pain and general health;

2. basic neurologic tests;

3. spine stabilization capabilities, including an overall *functional score*;

4. strength measures;

5. spinal range of motion (both cervical and lumbar); and

6. aerobic (MET) level.

PAIN AND GENERAL HEALTH

In this section, there are five parameters. The first is a pain rating, which is the patient's numerical rating of his or her pain that day, ranging from 0 to 10. *No pain* is 0, and *the worst pain imaginable* is 10, and can be represented on a visual analog scale, if needed. The next two numbers should represent the percentage of central spine pain versus radiating pain. It can represent cervical or lumbar problems. This can be a very helpful way of recording progress with eliminating radicular symptoms.

The last two parameters in this first section are the patient's body weight and a record of how much they are smoking. These are both areas where the therapist reinforces the physician's recommendations to the patient. Weight loss and smoking cessation are the two most common general health recommendations made to our spine patients. These parameters can help document the patient's general level of motivation in the program as well.

NEUROLOGIC SCREENS

Four neurologic screens were selected which can also be used as parameters of progress for the spine patient. We recommend several spine examination texts (see annotated bibliography), for those unfamiliar with these screens. We have found these to be very useful as well for use with the postoperative patient. Because of the limited space on the form, and the fact that we want the form to remain easy to read rapidly, we specify recording losses (abnormal findings) only. If everything is normal for a given category, writing either *normal* or *OK* can verify the fact that the tests were actually done.

The neurologic screens include:

1. *weakness,* referring to extremity motor loss;

2. *reflexes,* includes Achilles and patellar tendon for lumbar patients; biceps, triceps, and brachioradialis for cervical patients;

3. *straight leg raise* (SLR) for lower limb neural tension; and

4. *sensory testing* for the pertinent dermatomes for either lumbar or cervical patients.

Other applicable neurologic findings can be included in this section. For example, a positive femoral nerve tension test can be included in the SLR column. In the cervical patient with positive upper limb tension tests, the SLR slot may be replaced by *ULTT* for upper limb tension test. It is helpful to specify *median nerve,* for example, so that another therapist can test in just that position.

STABILIZATION TESTS

This section was one of the most difficult sections of consensus among our therapists because there is so little validity or reliability in strength testing. Assessing spine stabilization capability is even more difficult, because clear definitions of spine stabilization are not agreed upon. However, there are some commonly used tests of basic stabilization exercise performance that do not require equipment. The group finally agreed on these tests, but we are very open to suggestions for improvement in this area. The tests are a modified version of tests published by Saal (1991, 1992) at the San Francisco Spine Institute. Our modifications were mostly further clarification of the positioning, timing, and passing requirements for the tests. The description below is what we use for a Level I test. Levels II and III described by the Saal brothers proved to be too difficult for our more deconditioned general patient population, so we lowered requirements for these levels. To create level II and III tests, simply extend the time period for maintaining each of the exercises listed below.

The first two tests are of abdominal strength. Two tests are provided so that if the patient has cervical spine problems and cannot effectively perform abdominal curls without neck pain, the fully supported "dead bug" test can be substituted. The first test is three sets of ten abdominal curls, one straight and one oblique to each side, with no rest between sets. Hands may be behind the head, or crossed over the chest and the scapula must clear the floor or mat on each repetition. The three sets must be completed within one minute. The "dead bug" test starts in the supine position with arms and thighs pointed at the ceiling, at a right angle to the body, and knees bent to ninety degrees. Opposite arm and leg are lowered toward the floor without touching it, then returned to the starting position in a continuous motion as the other arm and leg extend. The arm and leg motions continue for one minute, requiring constant activity of the abdominals, as the *lumbar spine must not move.* To verify no movement of the lumbar spine, a partially inflated blood pressure cuff may be placed under the low back and should stay at the same reading. The patient can also balance a dowel rod across the abdomen to assess the steadiness of the spine during the arm and leg movements.

The next tests are of back extensor strength. Again, two tests are provided as the prone position can be painful for some postoperative fusion patients. If the patient is able, we encourage both tests, however, as the prone test is the best representation of back extensor function without contribution from hip movement. One minute of prone extension, with the upper body suspended horizontally while legs are secured, as described in the *Sorenson Test* (Moffroid et al. 1993), is the passing grade for Level I stabilization. Two minutes of continuous bridging (small motions of the hips up and down are allowed) is the Level I stabilization test for back and hip extensors. Again, balancing a dowel rod across the pelvis can assure maintenance of a constant back position.

Wall squats are the test for leg strength, with the subject standing with the back supported on the wall with hips and knees close to ninety degree angles for one minute (for Level I stabilization). Patients with knee or hip problems that prevent them from going this low on the wall can assume a slightly higher position on the wall, with the knee angle documented to keep the tests consistent from week to week.

Functional score is a composite score of capabilities to do five functional movements: stooping to the floor, reaching overhead, going from sitting to standing, going from sitting to lying, and rolling with the proper body mechanics. The descriptions and the point system are described in Saal's (1991) article. In Saal's test, two points are given if the activity is done with proper body mechanics without cuing, one point if cuing is required, and zero if it is still not done correctly, so a perfect functional score is ten.

STRENGTH TESTS

Grip strength is not only included for an upper extremity strength measure, but was also chosen because of its relation to overall body strength. Most clinics have grip strength dynamometers, even if they don't have other pieces of strength testing equipment. These readings are also helpful in the cases of cervical spine pathologies if motor loss is involved or suspected.

Grip strength will also be used to determine the rate of progression for weight lifting exercises, once the patient passes Level I stabilization and shows average or better MET level on aerobic testing.

Lifting tests are done using a box lift, waist to shoulder height, starting with ten pounds and lifting with proper mechanics fifteen to twenty repetitions in one minute. If these are done successfully, the weight may be increased in five pound increments to a maximum of twenty-five percent of the grip strength per week. Therefore, an individual having a thirty pound grip strength could not increase more than one five pound increment per week (two five pound increments, or ten pounds would be greater than twenty-five percent of thirty pounds of grip). An individual with forty pounds of grip could increase up to ten pounds per week. The box lift test is repeated lifting from floor to waist height.

We also recommend individuals with more than one hundred pounds of grip strength not advance more than twenty-five pounds per week. It may be necessary to limit this progression even more, for the safety of some patients.

SPINAL RANGE OF MOTION

The spinal range of motion is measured with inclinometers, if available. It is recommended that measurements are done in both cervical and lumbar spine areas to help identify concurrent problems, as well as to document consistency in the patient's performance. Details regarding the inclinometer measures are given in the previous chapter.

MET LEVEL

Any test measuring aerobic capacity can be used in this category. In our testing system, we use testing as specified in the *ACSM Guidelines for Exercise Testing and Prescription, 5th edition* (1995). Details and forms for testing are included in the next chapter. We chose to use

Physical Capacity Testing

Patient: ———————————— Physician: ———————————— DOI: ————

Diagnosis: ———— HT: ———— WT: ———— Employer / Job Title: ————

	/	/	/	/	/
Pain Rating					
% Pain Spine					
% Pain Ext.					
Weight					
Smoking (amt)					
Neuro Screen (losses only)					
Weakness					
Reflexes					
SLR test					
Sensory					
Stabilization					
Abs- diagonal					
Abs. dead bug					
Extensors- prone					
Ext.- slow bridge					
Wall squats					
Functional score					
Grip Strength	R L	R L	R L	R L	R L
Lifting Test: (15-20 reps in one minute) Progress in 5# increments to maximum per week of 25% of patients grip strength					
Cx: waist to sh. (wt)					
Lum: floor to waist (wt)					
ROM /Posture					
Cx. Flexion					
Cx. Extension					
Cx. Rotation	R L	R L	R L	R L	R L
Lum. Flexion					
Lum. Extension					
Lum. Lat. Flex	R L	R L	R L	R L	R L
Standing Posture	T L	T L	T L	T L	T L
MET level					
Walking/20 min.					
CV. test/grade					

Figure 9. Physical Capacities Test Form

MET levels as opposed to VO_2 values because MET level numbers are smaller, making categorization of patients simpler. Our therapist group decided that a minimal aerobic level should be attained prior to weight lifting. In this way, the patient would be at less risk of fatigue that could injure them during the strength training. The minimal aerobic level to allow strength testing or training was the *average* level for an individual's age group and gender. (See MET level charts in Chapter 4, Figure 13.)

Chapter Four

•••••••••••••••

Cardiovascular Testing Examples
for the Physical Capacities Test

In some cases, separate considerations must be made regarding aerobic testing on patients. There are times when the rest of the PCT can be done, but the patient may not be ready for a cardiovascular test. In other cases, a patient may have already demonstrated good stabilization capabilities, and may just need to work on aerobic level to regain the endurance to return to work or other activity. Periodic cardiovascular tests may be the only testing needed at that stage. Many clinicians are very comfortable with all of the testing on the PCT except for the cardiovascular testing. In general, clinics that deal primarily with orthopedic patients do not delve into this area often. For this reason, the cardiovascular tests are covered in this separate chapter. We have found that with good background information, clinicians can feel confident about performing safe submaximal cardiovascular tests. The information obtained from these tests is extremely valuable for fully understanding the patient's activity tolerances. If the aerobic level is low, fatigue may discourage or entirely prevent the patient from returning to normal activities.

We strongly recommend having a copy of the *ACSM Guidelines* (1995) in the clinic and train all exercise personnel in the testing and training precautions and rules. The ACSM has published several editions of these guidelines, always updating with new information, with several charts for quick reference. Information for this chapter has been gathered from the 4th and 5th editions (ACSM 1991; 1995). There are also several variations of testing which might better match a particular clinic's set-up, time frames with patients, and equipment. A very important section in all editions covers pretest screening of patients with definitions of relative and absolute contraindications.

The second page of the Physical Capacities test form is entitled *Submaximal Graded Exercise Test,* and is shown in Figure 10. We use this type of test for estimating the aerobic levels for many spine patients. We use metabolic equivalents (METs) as the units to express the aerobic levels because they represent a small range of numbers, making it easy to categorize patients quickly. MET levels also represent oxygen consumption (VO_2), but again with smaller numbers. (MET value is VO_2 divided by 3.5) MET levels can be very helpful in understanding the patient's true exercise tolerance. If the patient has a low MET level, they are very likely to fatigue quickly and may not benefit much, if at all from strength training. Aerobic training for endurance needs to be the first area addressed in a deconditioned patient.

The test we most commonly use for MET level estimation is the modified Balke Protocol, which is covered in detail in the *ACSM Guidelines* (1991). We have summarized the protocol in Figure 11. We have included a conversion chart in Figure 12 showing example aerobic levels (in METs) for various treadmill speeds and grades. The original Balke protocol specifies just one speed for the treadmill, but the modified Balke allows for other speeds, so these conversions are needed. The ACSM has more of these charts and formulas to make possible variations on these tests. They also have a conversion chart for several leisure activities and sports in terms of MET levels (ACSM 1991;1995). There are several other texts with similar charts available as well (Hoeger 1986; Skinner 1993).

Because spine patients cannot always tolerate the incline needed for the standard treadmill tests, an alternative test which looks only at distance covered over time can be used to estimate MET level. There are also conversion charts equating walking speed with MET levels, so a simple timed walk could be used with level surfaces. The most common tests are the Six Minute Walk test and the Twelve Minute Walk test (Skinner 1993). We use the PCT form to record times, speeds, elevations, and heart rates during these tests. Also, for those patients who cannot use heart rate to monitor level of exertion, a Borg Scale of perceived exertion is helpful (ACSM 1995; Skinner 1993). With the Borg scale, a visual analog scale, set using a 1-20 rating, is used. The numbers are arranged similarly to those on a thermometer with word descriptors about every third number ranging from *very, very light* (at level 7 on the Borg scale), through *somewhat hard,* to *very, very hard* (level 19). The patient describes how hard they are working, and the number associated with the descriptor tends to represent the heart rate when a zero is added to the end of the scale number.

We recommend choosing a minimum MET level by age and gender, using either the ACSM or the American Heart Association fitness charts and use that minimum as a standard to allow individuals to begin strength training. We have illustrated the American Heart Association chart in Figure 13, which we converted from VO_2 values for our categorization of patients (Hoeger 1986). We have chosen the *average* category as the minimum requirement to allow strength training for our spine patients, whether the patients are surgical or nonsurgical. They must be at the minimum MET level to help insure that they will not be injured simply due to fatigue when beginning strength training. Please recall also that the patients

Submaximal Graded Treadmill Exercise Test

Patient: _____   Predicted max HR: _____   Target HR: _____ (___%)

Age: _____   WT: _____   Medications: _____

Date / / / / /

Test #																				
	TM speed	% grade	HR	mets	TM speed	% grade	HR	mets	TM speed	% grade	HR	mets	TM speed	% grade	HR	mets	TM speed	% grade	HR	mets
Min 1																				
2																				
3																				
4																				
5																				
6																				
7																				
8																				
9																				
10																				
11																				
12																				
13																				
14																				
15																				

Reasons for stopping and comments: _____
_____

Test Date and #					Comments:
Results: Estimated MET Capacity					
VO2 MAX (ml/kg/min)					
Cardiovascular Classification (AHA)					
12 Min. Walk Test: DIS.:					
METS:					
Cardiovascular Classification (AHA):					

Figure 10. Submaximal Graded Treadmill Exercise Test Form

are required to pass the Level I spine stabilization screen, which would demonstrate that they have adequate foundation strength to safely start lifting training.

Both the ACSM and Skinner texts fully explain exercise testing and interpretation of the "normal" population with comparison to that for people with all types of complications, ranging from musculoskeletal, to cardiovascular, to systemic disorders such as diabetes. There is a chapter in Skinner (1993) on testing and training for patients with low back pain which reviews the current research in this area.

Figure 11. Modified Balke Treadmill Test Protocol

—modified and adapted from the *ACSM Guidelines* (1991, 1995)

1. If there is any doubt about the patient's readiness or safety for this test, do not perform the test.

2. Record the patient's age and calculate *predicted maximal heart rate* (max. HR) by subtracting the patient's age from 220.

3. Calculate the target heart rate (target HR), the maximal rate allowed during the test, which can range from sixty-five percent, for a deconditioned patient, to eighty percent for a conditioned patient. Enter the heart rate value and the percentage you used to calculate it at the top of the form.

4. Explain the test to the patient thoroughly before beginning testing. Be sure the patient understands all signs of overexertion and the importance of their feedback to stop the test if needed. It is best to do this test using a heart rate monitor.

5. The test is done at a set speed. For most tests, elevation is increased every two minutes. Record treadmill speed, percentage elevation, and heart rate at the end of each minute of the test.

6. Continue the test until the patient reaches the target heart rate, or complains of shortness of breath, dizziness, chest pain, or extreme fatigue.

7. Complete the fourth column of the recording chart, the MET levels associated with walking at each speed and elevation.

8. Using graph paper (or a computer program set up for this), graph the heart rates versus the MET levels for every two minutes of the test. Make a line of "best fit" to the graphed points. Draw a line from the maximal heart rate to the line of best fit. The estimated maximal MET level can be read on the perpendicular drawn from this point to the MET level axis.

Figure 12. Sample Treadmill Test Values (ACSM 1991)

2.5 miles per hour

0% grade	=	2.9 METs
2.5% grade	=	3.8 METs
5.0% grade	=	4.6 METs
7.5% grade	=	5.2 METs
10.0% grade	=	6.3 METs

3.0 miles per hour

0% grade	=	3.3 METs
2.5% grade	=	4.3 METs
5.0% grade	=	5.4 METs
7.5% grade	=	6.3 METs
10.0% grade	=	7.4 METs

(figure cont. on nest page)

4.0 miles per hour

0% grade	=	4.0 METs
2.5% grade	=	5.4 METs
5.0% grade	=	6.8 METs
7.5% grade	=	8.1 METs
10.0% grade	=	9.2 METs

Figure 13. American Heart Association (AHA) Norms for MET level

(Hoeger 1986, with reference to American Heart Association Exercise Testing and Training of Apparently Healthy Individuals: A Handbook for Physicians.)

AGE	LOW	FAIR	AVERAGE	GOOD	HIGH
			WOMEN		
20-29	< 6.8	6.8-8.6	8.7-10.5	10.6-13.7	13.8+
30-39	< 5.7	5.7-7.7	7.8-9.4	9.5-12.6	12.7+
40-49	< 4.9	4.9-6.6	6.7-8.6	8.7-11.7	11.8+
50-59	< 4.3	4.3-5.7	5.8-7.7	7.8-10.6	10.7+
60-69	< 3.7	3.7-4.9	5.0-6.6	6.7-9.9	10.0+
			MEN		
20-29	< 7.1	7.1-9.4	9.5-12.2	12.3-14.9	15.0+
30-39	< 6.6	6.6-8.6	8.7-10.6	10.7-13.7	13.8+
40-49	< 5.7	5.7-7.4	7.5-10.0	10.1-12.6	12.7+
50-59	< 5.1	5.1-6.9	7.0-9.4	9.5-12.0	12.1+
60-69	< 4.6	4.6-6.3	6.4-8.6	8.7-11.4	11.5+

Chapter Five

•..•❶••••••••

In-Patient Postsurgical Protocols

In the current healthcare environment, the surgical spine patient is not in the hospital for more than a day or so in most cases. Many patients also have surgery on an out-patient basis. There is not time in a typical hospital stay for therapy to take place, other than a one-time visit, in most cases. Often, the one-time visit is not possible either. However, these protocols were designed when patients were in the hospital for several days at least. We originally thought of discarding the protocols and then decided they could be helpful for therapists caring for the postsurgical patient in a longterm health care facility or in home health. In either of these situations, the surgeon may opt to have the patient start therapy early, especially for restoring the patient's self-care abilities. These protocols, found in Figures 15 and 16, can help the patient recruit needed musculature and reinforce an activity habit, as opposed to a fear of movement altogether. In addition, we are optimistic about the future therapist's role of increased involvement with the surgical patient, when in-patient physical therapy is a standing order for all patients.

We recommend these protocols beginning the first or second day after surgery, depending on the patient's capability to do the movements. The patient can follow these programs until they are

LUMBAR EARLY POSTOPERATIVE EVALUATION Form (within first 2 weeks)

Patient name_____DOB_____

Date of evaluation_____Date of procedure_____

SURGERY (levels & type) _____

❑ **Spine Inspection:** L-spine contour:_____steps_____irreg. soft tissue;
incision description & location_____;
discoloration_____; drainage_____; swelling_____;
other:_____.

❑ Posture:____kyphosis (norm, xs); _____lordosis (norm, xs) ; _____R / L lat shift.
   Asymmetries L/R: Head_____; shoulders_____; iliac_____; PSIS_____;
      legs/feet___/_____; other_____.
      Sagittal deviations: head/shoulders_____; trunk_____; pelvis_____.

❑ **Neurologic Screen**
❑DTR's_____❑ SLR_____❑ Femoral Nv._____
❑SENSORY_____
❑MOTOR_____
❑ Babinski _____; Clonus_____; other_____
❑ Foot Pulses:_____

❑ Gait: _____normal; _____Deviation:_____. Daily walking distance/time_____.
❑ FUNCTIONAL MOBILITY: log roll_____;supine/sit_____; sit/stand_____;
standing balance_____; self care/bathroom_____; partial squat supported_____;
reach overhead_____.   (KEY: OK, U=unable, NI= needs improvement)
❑ Pertinent Lower Extremity ROM limitations:

PLAN: (include each checked item):

_____therapist _____ dictated

Figure 14. Lumbar Early Postsurgical Evaluation Form
(within first 2 weeks)

evaluated later as out-patients when they would progress to the regular out-patient protocols outlined in Chapters 6 and 7. For younger or more active patients with less complicated surgeries, these protocols would apply only for the first week or two, if the patient could progress into more advanced exercises with supervision.

The emphasis in the very early postoperative stages should be on patient education. It is up to the therapist to individualize care at this stage. Helping the patient identify the best means of posture, positioning, and support to minimize discomfort and facilitate function should be a primary goal. Unnecessary fears can be minimized. When the therapist has adequate information about the surgery, with the surgeon's agreement, details surrounding the surgery can be discussed. All of these steps can help the patient be a more active participant in the rehabilitation process.

Full postsurgical evaluation as described in Chapter 2 will probably not be possible or appropriate in the first days after surgery. The neurologic tests are important and should be done, to the extent that pain allows. Full muscle testing may need to be deferred. Postural assessment, incision inspection, and capabilities for basic activities of daily living can be very helpful at this stage too. An early postsurgical evaluation form example is shown in Figure 14.

Figure 15. In-patient Postsurgical Lumbar Protocol for Nonfusion Surgeries:

laminectomy, decompressive laminectomy, microdiscectomy, endoscopic procedures

REHABILITATION GOALS

1. Evaluate patient with regard to neurologic screens, incision status, postural assessment, basic activities of daily living

2. Educate patient regarding surgical procedure to the extent allowable by referring physician. Discuss postsurgical restrictions and approximate time frames, which usually extend until first physician's postsurgical office visit (from four to six weeks after surgery).

3. Establish best means of posture, positioning, and support of the spine to minimize discomfort and to facilitate spine stabilization.

4. Initiate early spine rehabilitation with attention to symptom changes and additional precautions specified by the surgeon. Gradual mobility will be the general goal, but nothing should produce or increase radiating leg pain.

REHABILITATION PROGRAM

1. Evaluate using early postsurgical evaluation form (Figure 14).

2. Identify the most important needs based on the evaluation, in case therapy visits are limited to one or two. Set up a walking program for the patient.

3. Review physician's specific postoperative restrictions: for example, no bending, no lifting more than five pounds, no twisting, etc. Be sure to address driving and sex, the two areas patients will most often save to discuss with their therapist. Use videotaped or printed instructions described in Chapter 6, Figure 18.

4. Review posture, positioning, and support. Instruct in use of brace, if ordered. Instruct in needed body mechanics found in the postoperative evaluation.

5. Begin spine stabilization exercise with the following guidelines. (See Chapter 10 for more details.)

    a. Abdominal and back extensor muscle recruitment:

- Do isometrics or small range movements only, in pain free positions, for the first two weeks (Figure 30, #1; Figure 31, #1 and #2).
- If there is no leg pain after two weeks of isometrics, spinal motion can occur with exercise. (Fig. 40)

- The back should be fully supported; may use pillow(s) for added support.
  b. Very gentle work on neural mobility, maintaining neutral spine, and not provoking *any* symptoms:
    - Calf pumping and ankle mobility are key, and a good starting point for more proximal work.
    - Posterior thigh stretching is done, working hip and knee separately at first, in a supine position with other knee flexed (Figure 40, #5).
    - Anterior thigh stretching is done, in sidelying or prone, avoiding twisting or bending of the spine (Figure 35).
  c. Upper extremity exercise and cervical ROM may be integrated into this regimen, as long as the patient is able to maintain neutral spine positioning, and avoids aggravating symptoms (Figures 46 and 47).
  d. Functional activity practice may begin if it can be done without leg pain (Figure 33).

Figure 16. In-patient Postsurgical Lumbar Protocol for Fusion Surgeries

REHABILITATION GOALS

1. Evaluate patient with regard to neurologic screens, incision status, postural assessment, basic activities of daily living.

2. Educate patient regarding surgical procedure to the extent allowable by referring physician. If possible, discuss type and location of fusion and hardware used (if applicable) to help orient the patient. Discuss postsurgical restrictions. Review time frame: two to four months of rehabilitation may be necessary.

3. Establish best means of posture, positioning, and support of the spine to minimize discomfort and to facilitate spine stabilization.

4. Initiate early spine rehabilitation with attention to symptom changes and additional precautions specified by the surgeon. Early emphasis after fusion is on restoring muscular support to the low back in neutral positions of the spine.

REHABILITATION PROGRAM

1. Evaluate using early postsurgical evaluation form (Figure 14).

2. Identify most important needs based on the evaluation, in case therapy visits are limited to one or two. First, emphasize the need to stabilize following a fusion (for several weeks; period of time may vary with surgeon), then establish mobility.

3. Review physician's specific postoperative restrictions: for example, no bending, no lifting more than five pounds, no twisting, etc. Be sure to address driving and sex, the two areas patients will most often save to discuss with their therapist. Use video tape instructions described in Chapter 7 and patient instructions found in Chapter 6 and 7 (Figures 18, 21, and 22).

4. Stress the importance of frequent walking, gently increasing distance. Set distance goal for each check-up with the physician: for example, two miles by six week postsurgical office visit.

5. Review posture, positioning, and support. Instruct in use of brace, if ordered. Instruct in body mechanics if identified in the postoperative evaluation as needing improvement.

6. Begin spine stabilization exercise with the following guidelines:

    a. Abdominal and back extensor muscle recruitment:
- Isometrics and small range movements only are done, in pain free positions (Figure 30, #1; Figure 31, #2; Figure 43).
- The back is fully supported; may use pillow(s) for added support.

b. Very gentle work should start with neural mobility, maintaining neutral spine, and not provoking *any* symptoms. Following fusions, patients may only be able to move in a small part of the exercise range. It is helpful to record the pain-free range possible and use it as a parameter for progress.

- Calf pumping and ankle mobility are key, and a good starting point for more proximal work.
- Posterior thigh stretching is done, working hip and knee separately at first, in a supine position with other knee flexed (Figure 34).
- Anterior thigh stretching is done, in sidelying or prone, avoiding twisting or bending of the spine (Figure 35).

c. Upper extremity exercise and cervical ROM may be integrated into this regimen, as long as the patient is able to maintain neutral spine positioning, and avoids aggravating symptoms. Also patients with fusions often respond best by doing the upper extremity work lying down with knees bent. Some examples of upper body exercise are found in Chapter 10 (Figures 46 and 47).

Chapter Six

•••••••••••••

Managing Patients Following Lumbar Surgeries Without Fusion

For the most part, the earlier the patient with non-fusion surgery can be seen, the better. The two most common complicating factors with this surgery, adherent nerve root and reherniation of the disc, could be lessened with early work in therapy (Poole 1997). The disc must be protected in the first several days, and the patient is more likely to understand how to do this with some guidance. With regard to the adherent nerve, early gentle mobility, *with precautions,* can help decrease scar tissue, at least theoretically. The best case scenario is seeing the patient in the hospital with the protocols described in the previous chapter. Logistics in the current health care environment often make the in-patient visit impossible. The next best alternative is to see the patient within the first two weeks of the surgery. Both Figure 15 and the first part of Figure 17 describe the rehabilitation goals and protocol for seeing patients in this time frame.

Unfortunately, most patients are sent home with driving restrictions for 4 to 6 weeks, which usually limits their access to out-patient rehabilitation. The patients are usually too healthy to receive home health. We have had the best luck seeing people early by coordinating their physical therapy visit with the visit for suture removal. Many problems are circumvented in a timely manner by seeing the patient at least once this early. Of course, if there are problems with wound healing, or increases in symptoms following the surgery, therapy is deferred. If feasible, the one visit at ten days to two weeks following surgery at the suture removal visit can be used to assign the patient some basic exercises to do at home, and to strongly reinforce proper postures, positioning, and support. The patient can keep in touch by phone if they have any problems between then and starting therapy another week or two later. Figure 17 also gives rehabilitation goals and protocol for seeing patients from two to six weeks after surgery.

The patient instructions in Figure 18 were written to instruct the patient for the first six weeks following surgery. Because of our setting, where many patients live a long distance from us, we often are limited to the six week checkup with the surgeon as our first therapy visit. Again, earlier visits have been a challenge for us to orchestrate. So the best we can do is try to tailor our programs for patients with limited visits to give them the most education possible, and then become their contact person answering questions on activities and exercise.

We designed a video tape called *The First Six Weeks* (Spine Care Associates of Tyler 1994) for our clinic and physicians that we serve, describing generic precautions and body mechanics which are common to most lumbar and cervical surgeries. Topics on this tape include getting in and out of a bed, chair, or car, alternatives to bending for going toward the floor, low area, or using a sink, and ways to sit and rest with back support. Walking and activities that have been approved by the surgeon are encouraged. A short section on signs of infection, dressings, and medications is included. We then supplement the tape with the Patient Instructions on the specific surgery. If the patient will be attending therapy in an outlying area, we send along a sheet of therapist notes with more information on the surgery and recommendations for prioritizing therapy. (See Figure 19.) We are fortunate to have a congenial group of therapists that are not offended by these instructions and will contact us if they run into problems in the patient's care.

Figure 17. Postsurgical Lumbar Protocol for Nonfusion Surgeries

laminectomy, discectomy, decompressive laminectomy, microscopic and endoscopic procedures

REHABILITATION GOALS, 0-2 WEEKS

1. Instruct in movement precautions and activity limitations, as outlined in patient instruction sheet for each specific surgery.

2. Increase lower extremity function (only with neutral spine maintained), and minimize any radiating symptoms.

3. Release soft tissue restrictions/muscle spasms, again maintaining neutral spine position.

4. Introduce/reintroduce spine stabilization, especially identifying neutral spine position and using muscular bracing. Level I exercises may begin at any point the patient can perform the movements without pain.

5. Impose a five pound lifting limit to allow for healing time before loading.

6. Initiate cardiovascular retraining.

REHABILITATION PROGRAM, 0-2 WEEKS

1. Progress walking within patient tolerance, at least twice a day.

2. Continue spine stabilization exercises as specified during the hospital stay or before.

3. Start neural mobility work for lower extremities as specified while in hospital or presurgically.

4. Instruct in functional activity as per patient instruction sheet (i.e. log roll out of bed, proper up and down from chair and floor).

5. Instruct patient in home care for soft tissue (lumbar roll, ice packs, etc.).

REHABILITATION GOALS, 2-6 WEEKS

Formal physical therapy may start at any point during this time frame. The patient will benefit most if symptoms are manageable and/or decreasing at the time they are beginning therapy.

1. Reinforce body mechanics and neutral spine for protection during activities. First priority of this time frame is producing muscular stabilization of the spine. Try to complete Level I stabilization during the first six weeks.

2. Restore functional range of motion to the lumbar spine, with careful attention not to reproduce any radiating symptoms.

3. Release soft tissue restrictions/muscle spasms. Watch incision area.

4. Progress cardiovascular training.

5. Initiate strength training as soon as Level I stabilization screens are passed.

REHABILITATION PROGRAM, 2-6 WEEKS

1. Progress walking to two miles (one mile in morning and one in evening).

2. Begin mobilization and active range of motion exercises for the spine.

3. Increase lifting limit to ten pounds, but it remains at that level until patient can pass Level I spine stabilization screens.

4. Instruct in Level I spine stabilization emphasizing neutral spine in position of greatest comfort, with flexion or extension bias exercise as needed to avoid position sensitivities and to reinforce structural changes made with the surgery.

5. Begin Physical Capacities Tests (PCT) at week four of therapy if possible, and do them every two weeks thereafter to quantify parameters of progress.

6. Train in body mechanics and functional movement.

7. Limit strength training to elastic resistance and decompression pulleys or light weights with back fully supported, unless patient passes Level I PCT (i.e. Level I spine stabilization screens, has above average MET level and generally has seventy-five percent normal lumbar range of motion. See Chapter 3 for details).

8. Carry out initial Functional Capacity Evaluation (FCE) for determination of readiness for work hardening, or return to work for lighter jobs. This may be done at six weeks, if patient is able to complete all of the above program components.

Note: Patients often do not have any exposure to rehabilitation until six weeks or more after surgery. A first-time patient should begin the protocol with the 0-2 week program and progress through as they are able to complete the steps. Sometimes these delayed patients can progress rapidly and require only a few weeks to reach FCE level. However, many times the patient will require substantially more than six weeks to be able to accomplish all steps. It is very important to document the level of deconditioning at the initial visit to justify the extra time. Then with PCTs every two weeks, continual progress can be documented in a way that should classify the patient's case as exceptional and warrants more time.

Figure 18. Patient Instructions

Lumbar Laminectomy, Discectomy, or Microdiscectomy Surgery

1. No lifting over ten pounds until your six week postop follow-up, unless your surgeon tells you otherwise. If you are sent to physical therapy before your six week checkup, the therapist may clear you to lift more before six weeks.

2. No bending, no stooping, and no twisting for the first four weeks. Activities and movements should not be painful under any circumstance.

3. Use good body mechanics when changing positions. When getting up from lying down, always log roll to your side *first*. Then sit up by pushing up from your side.

4. Support the low back with a pillow whenever you sit. Avoid prolonged sitting. Thirty minutes should be the maximum amount of time seated.

5. Preferred sleeping positions: on your side with knees bent and a pillow between them, or on your back with pillows under your knees.

6. It is best to avoid sex the first two weeks, or if pain increases significantly after the surgery. Once you resume sex, you still must observe the lifting and bending restrictions listed above. Sidelying is the safest approach.

7. Usually no driving is allowed for the first six weeks, especially if you are still having any leg pain.

8. Return to work release *must* be given by your physician before you return to work.

9. The first few weeks after surgery, walk as much as possible, and do only exercises given by the physical therapist.

10. It is helpful to lie on your stomach on a pillow which will take the curve out of your low back. Apply ice for fifteen to twenty minutes. This can be done several times per day as needed to reduce pain or swelling.

11. In order to help you move more easily when you first get up from lying down, do the following. Turn onto your back, and bend your knees as much as possible comfortably with both feet flat on the bed. Then, *gently*, rock your knees from side to side only moving about an inch in each direction at a pace of about two per second. Try to do this for two to three minutes. It will help circulation and be a "warm-up" which will allow you to move more easily afterward. Rocking in a rocking chair can help in the same way. Always rock *gently*.

Please call the physical therapy department if you have any questions.

Figure 19. Therapist Notes for Nonfusion Lumbar Surgeries

lumbar laminectomy, discectomy, decompression
laminectomy, microendoscopic discectomy

1. The purpose of these surgeries can vary depending on the presurgical diagnosis. With spinal stenosis, decompression laminectomy can involve the largest amounts of lamina removed, with higher risk of instability or scar tissue adherence. An uncomplicated HNP can often be resolved with very little lamina removed.

It is very important to know the presurgical diagnosis, and it also helps considerably to have an operative report.

2. Patients with less invasive surgeries can often benefit from early rehabilitation. The protocols are written to suggest safe movements for the patient starting early rehabilitation (at one to two weeks following surgery), under certain conditions: a) radiating pain is under control; b) the wound is healing well; and c) the patient is not markedly position or pressure sensitive.

3. Early therapy emphasis should be on:

   a. spine stabilization, with focus on maximizing recruitment of trunk muscles;

   b. attention to position and weight bearing sensitivities, and tailoring exercises accordingly;

   c. attention to incision and possible use of modalities and/or soft tissue mobilization to decrease scar tissue complications;

   d. frequent neurologic checks, and work on neural mobility.

4. Active range of motion exercises for the spine must be done using disc precautions. Therefore, reinforce avoidance of unsupported forward bending, twisting, or motion that reproduces leg pain.

5. Exercise program should follow spine stabilization principles. First, start with supported small movements; second, increase the range of extremity movement; and then decrease the trunk support. Patients are instructed to avoid lifting until they are able to pass Level I spine stabilization.

6. It is important to initiate cardiovascular training early in the treatment program to help build and restore fatigue resistance, especially in those patients who test with fair or poor MET level. Test MET level every two weeks to determine patient progress.

Chapter Seven

•••••●●•••••••••••

Managing Patients
Following Lumbar Fusion

This protocol was developed for patients to have their first post-surgical evaluation for rehabilitation at six weeks following the surgery. This was done mostly for logistics, as the patients in our practice are not generally seen by the surgeon until this time, and so we often do not see them until that point. With fusions, most surgeons are hesitant to send patients to therapy until they have seen the patient for that first visit, and often, do not do so until the patient has had the six week postsurgical x-rays. Good preoperative instruction and in-hospital instruction can give the patient guidelines for the first six weeks. Videotaped instructions of do's and don'ts as well as a good description of any red flag conditions (i.e. signs of infection, significant changes in symptoms) can help reassure the patient, and also start the recovery process with the best mechanical advantages. Our *First Six Weeks* videotape, published by SpineCare of Tyler, Texas in 1994, was made to address these areas. Written instructions can serve the same purpose, and we have presented some at the end of this chapter (Figure 21 and 22).

The therapy that is selected at the time of the six week postsurgical evaluation will vary considerably between individuals and will be based on evaluation findings. For fusion patients, the use of functional loss characteristics (see Chapter 1, Figure 1) is very helpful in establishing priorities for the rehabilitation program, if the patient is still very symptomatic. The guidelines in the protocol are in time frames for best case scenarios, for patients who have little pain with capabilities to progress with an exercise program. Others must have lengthened time frames.

Lumbar fusion patients can experience all of the mechanical effects noted in the nonfusion chapter, but also have the added factor of architectural change. The fused levels change the nature of the motion at the other segments and conceivably change some of the adjacent muscle functions. Some previously mobile muscle attachments may have become fixed. With interbody fusions, the intervertebral space is often increased considerably. With more than one level fused, the degree of the potential mechanical impact, via increased vertical force, increases. These are our clinical observations and our theories regarding cause.

Anterior approach surgeries appear to differ from posterior approach surgeries in mechanical tendencies. For example, anterior surgeries may produce a tendency toward increasing lumbar lordosis, and at times, problems with mechanical pain from resulting forces on the facets. The patient with anterior approach may have more trouble tolerating upright at first, and may be helped by a brace designed to reduce the lordosis. Posterior approach surgeries can move toward a "flat back" posture, and may have difficulties learning to recruit the back extensor musculature after surgery. The lack of ability to recruit back extensors with other lumbar pathologies has been documented in the past (Hides et al. 1996), and the surgery can produce another factor that must be overcome to restore function. Surgeries using both approaches, the "360" surgeries, sometimes appear to cancel out some of the anterior versus posterior mechanical effects. The issue of muscle recruitment in the postoperative spinal fusion patient needs to be studied further.

Neurologic considerations following spinal fusion should include not only the monitoring of neurologic signs, but also the quality of motor control of the operated area. Muscle recruitment for recovery of support strength to the lower trunk may require extra time and facilitation techniques to be sure that recovery is maximal (Gill and Callaghan 1998). Studies have shown proprioception changes with lumbar spine problems (Hides et al. 1996). Also, the consideration of neural mobility is important throughout the care of the spine patient (Kornberg and McCarthy 1992). Postfusion surgery should be no exception.

Figure 20 provides a protocol for all fusion surgeries. This protocol represents a general progression for all fusion surgeries, with specific adaptations for anterior and posterior approach fusions, described in Therapist notes (Figure 23 and 24). Time frames may be adjusted on a case by case basis by the surgeon. Our surgeons felt that time frames in general should be the same whether or not the patient has fusion with hardware. All time frames refer to number of weeks after date of surgery.

Figure 20. Protocol for Lumbar Fusion Surgeries

REHABILITATION GOALS, 1-6 weeks: (may be achieved with presurgical visit, in-patient hospital visit; or postsurgical phone follow-up)

1. Be sure patient knows home exercise (mostly isometric) and beginning muscle recruitment for stabilization.

2. Remind patient to continue to observe precautions as instructed in the hospital (and demonstrated on *The First Six Weeks* video)

3. Increase lower extremity function; work on restoration of any strength losses, mostly with walking and calf pumping only.

4. Reinforce use of corset or brace. Reevaluate effectiveness of brace.

5. Reinforce five pound lifting limit until therapy begins.

6. Initiate home walking program, trying to increase distance to one to two miles by six week checkup with the surgeon.

REHABILITATION PROGRAM, 1-6 WEEKS

Refer to Chapter 5, Figure 16 for home exercise program to be taught either presurgically, in hospital, or at suture removal visit. All exercises are fully supported and neutral spine is strictly maintained. Gentle neural mobilization is included for the lower extremities to avoid adherent nerve root.

REHABILITATION GOALS, FROM THERAPY EVALUATION
TO 12 WEEKS AFTER SURGERY: (In cases where patients are doing very well, therapy may begin at 3 or 4 weeks postsurgically.)

1. Progress spine stabilization through fully supported exercise to upright exercise and then involve balance. Emphasize correct muscle recruitment.

2. Progress cardiovascular conditioning to augment other conditioning effort, and work on restoring or improving fatigue resistance.

3. Determine mechanical means of pain control for the patient using physical agents, positioning, support, or peripheral movements, as needed.

4. Progress lifting limit once patient is able to pass Level I spine stabilization screens and has adequate MET level on Physical Capacities Test.

5. Release soft tissue restrictions/muscle spasms.

6. Reinforce proper posture and body mechanics for all activities of daily living (ADLs). Prepare to wean from brace, if applicable.

REHABILITATION PROGRAM, THERAPY EVALUATION TO 12 WEEKS:

1. Begin Level I spine stabilization exercises, progressing to Level II, as soon as Level I screens are passed.

2. Progress aerobic program in intensity and/or duration to improve aerobic level and achieve at least three miles/day walking distance by twelve weeks.

3. Identify mechanical problems from therapy evaluation and address each in therapy program with positioning or movement if possible. Use physical agents or manual therapy to help minimize soft tissue restrictions and muscle spasms.

4. Include motor control considerations in the treatment program. Check for correct muscle recruitment and integrate coordination and quality of movement in the exercise.

5. Instruct proper body mechanics and postures for patient's ADLs.

6. Continue with neural mobilization and attention to lower extremity flexibility.

7. Begin periodic interim testing to assess progress, using the *Physical Capacities Test (PCT)* format, about every two weeks throughout the formal therapy.

REHABILITATION GOALS, 12-18 weeks following surgery, or through next six weeks of therapy.

(Note: Patients who are able to complete all steps from the 6-12 week protocol stage may advance to this stage sooner. Some patients may also require more than 6 weeks at the previous stage.)

1. Continue to maximize soft tissue function and mobility.

2. Seek continued improvement in muscle balance through the lower quarter, and minimize or eliminate radiating symptoms.

3. Maximize MET level. Work toward "average" to "good" level on AHA chart.

4. Restore needed lifting and strength capacity for return to work or entry into work hardening.

5. Maximize trunk strength and capability to isolate abdominals, back extensors, and hip musculature (for dynamic spine stabilization).

6. Continue to reinforce body mechanics and maintaining neutral spine throughout all conditioning exercise.

REHABILITATION PROGRAM, 12-18 WEEKS

1. Work on specific stretching and soft tissue/joint mobilization to maximize function in adjacent areas, such as thoracic spine, hips, and pelvis.

2. Continue spine stabilization exercise, emphasizing more upright posture and balance/coordination challenges, once Level I screens are passed on PCT.

3. Begin strength training, starting with decompression weights, and then introducing functional lifting (i.e. floor to waist and waist to shoulder).

4. Continue progress with cardiovascular conditioning.

5. Follow with FCE and work hardening, if needed.

Figure 21. Patient Instructions

*Anterior Approach Lumbar Fusion Surgeries
with or without Cage Implants*

1. Watch *The First Six Weeks* video and follow all advice.

2. Support the low back, at least with a soft pillow, whenever you sit. Do not sit without a slight sensation of pressure into your low back from the support.

3. Practice the basic stabilization exercises, a few reps at a time, several times a day. Remember, you are reprogramming the muscles to work with the new mechanics of the fusion. Some of the vertebrae in your low back that used to move are now in a fixed position. Do everything you can to let them heal in a good position (by learning to hold a good neutral spine) and to allow the muscles to start working as soon as possible in their new jobs.

4. Do not lift more than ten pounds until you are told otherwise after your six week checkup with the doctor and therapist. You will still have a lifting limit for a while after that, although you may be allowed to increase it some.

5. Be constantly aware of your posture. Your head needs to be right over your shoulders, shoulders back, and abdomen tight. Wear your brace if instructed by your surgeon.

6. It is best to avoid sex the first two weeks, or if pain increases significantly after the surgery. Once you resume sex, you still must observe the lifting and bending restrictions listed above and wear your brace. Sidelying is the safest approach.

7. Preferred sleeping positions: on your side with knees bent and a pillow between them, or on your back with pillows under your knees. Some patients obtain relief from wearing a brace at night, loosened slightly.

8. Whenever you get up from lying down, *always* log roll to your side first. Slide your legs to the side of the bed and drop your feet over, sitting up from your side.

9. The abdominals can be very stubborn in return function. The abdominal muscles are very weak in many individuals anyway, and the surgical incision often makes them even weaker. You can avoid this problem by making a concentrated effort to work these muscles frequently. Contract your abdominals with all of your exercises while placing one hand over your incision to see if you can activate the muscles there. Deep breathing helps work the abdominals when you tighten your abdomen as you breathe out.

10. You will be seen by the therapist on the day of your six week checkup with the doctor, unless you hear otherwise from our office. (Some people need to start sooner.) You must have appointments to see both the therapist and the doctor. If you do not have these appointments, please notify our office at (phone number): _____.

11. Please feel free to contact the therapist at (phone number): _____. We will return your call as soon as possible.

Figure 22. Patient Instructions:

Posterior Approach Lumbar Fusion Surgeries with or without Cage Implants and/or Pedicle Screws, or "360" Fusion Surgeries

1. Watch *The First Six Weeks* video and follow all advice.

2. Support the low back, at least with a soft pillow, whenever you sit. Do not sit without a slight sensation of pressure into your low back from the support.

3. Practice the basic stabilization exercises, a few reps at a time, several times a day. Remember, you are reprogramming the muscles to work with the new mechanics of the fusion. Some of the vertebrae in your low back that used to move are now in a fixed position. You want to do everything you can to let them heal in a good position (by learning to hold a good neutral spine) and to allow the muscles to start working as soon as possible in their new jobs.

4. Do not lift more than ten pounds until you are told otherwise after your six week checkup with the doctor and therapist. You will still have a lifting limit for a while after that, although you may be allowed to increase it some.

5. Be constantly aware of your posture. Your head needs to be right over your shoulders, shoulders back, and abdomen tight. Wear your brace if instructed by your surgeon.

6. It is best to avoid sex the first two weeks, or if pain increases significantly after the surgery. Once you resume sex, you still must observe the lifting and bending restrictions listed above and wear your brace. Sidelying is the safest approach.

7. Preferred sleeping positions: on your side with knees bent and a pillow between them, or on your back with pillows under your knees. Some patients obtain relief from wearing a brace at night, loosened slightly.

8. Whenever you get up from lying down, *always* log roll to your side first. Slide your legs to the side of the bed and drop your feet over, sitting up from your side.

9. The back muscles will tend to tighten and at times the low back will flatten. It is very important to maintain a slight arch in

your back to help reduce the pressure on the lower vertebrae. You will also have to relearn how to contract your abdominal muscles and back muscles. Your therapists will go over this with you and then you should *practice* several times a day. If you have trouble tolerating upright position (either sitting or standing), you may need a brace.

10. The "wall squat" exercise is safe to begin at any time and can be done in or out of your brace. Its a very effective lower body strengthener that will also help you get up and down from sitting and from the floor. It is important that the therapist watch you do this the first time to make sure you are doing it safely. Note: it is very important that your knees do not go in front of your feet and that your hips stay above the knees.

11. Your first therapy evaluation should be on the day of your six week checkup with the doctor, in most cases. For out-of-town patients seeing local therapists: have the therapist contact us for protocol information at (phone number):

_____.

12. Please feel free to contact the therapist at the above number phone number, or at (phone number): _____.

Figure 23. Therapist Notes
for Anterior Lumbar Fusion Surgeries

In addition *to postsurgical therapy protocol for lumbar fusion surgeries.*

1. The purpose of this surgery is usually to replace painful degenerated or internally disrupted discs. The surgery can also be done to repair a ruptured disc if the rupture is extensive or if instability is present. The BAK or cage implants afford more stability than most fusion devices because they take up most of the intervertebral space and do so with an expansion force into the space.

2. It is very important to know which levels were fused, and this information should arrive on the therapy prescription. The cage implants are perforated titanium that go in the disc space, then are packed with bone shavings and/or bone morphogenic protein. The vertebral bone should then grow through the cage to secure the fusion. The cages generally will increase the intervertebral space at that level and are more secure than bone plugs, but, they may create a constant stretch on previously lax ligaments and tendons, and possibly increase vertical forces on the adjacent vertebrae.

3. If the patient is having less pain following the surgery, early therapy is very helpful. Isometric trunk work with the therapist monitoring control of the muscles is a first step. Basic stabilization must be reviewed as the mechanics of neutral spine change a lot following the surgery. The fusion may create the impression that the patient can stabilize their spine easily, so it is important to watch and palpate for muscular control. Abdominals are the most difficult muscles to recruit, and should be an area of emphasis in every program. Obliques can often be recruited first, but need to be done with minimal trunk motion.

4. Measure and monitor posture as anterior approach surgeries often tend to have an increasing lordosis as the back extensors adaptively shorten after surgery and often overpower the weakened and usually overstretched abdominals. If you notice a changing posture, and especially if it is accompanied by increasing backache, a lumbosacral brace may help. Depending on the size of the patient you may opt for semirigid, or simply elastic. In some cases even rigid TLSO is appropriate, but only if you have consulted the physician.

5. Often flexion-biased aerobic exercise such as the bicycle or recumbent stepper (*not* upright) is best for these patients. If they can walk without increasing back or leg pain, walking is okay. The pool is great if you have it, but monitor the patient's heart rate to be sure the exercise is aerobic. We believe a good aerobic progression can

help patients achieve better early pain control and also, of course, minimize weight gain. Low aerobic levels also cause the patients to fatigue before they can benefit from other conditioning attempts, so this must be addressed as early as possible.

6. Manual therapy can often help facilitate exercise progression, or at least we think it can, based on our observations of these patients so far. Assisted hip stretching and T-spine mobilization with strict attention to maintaining neutral lumbar spine is often helpful. Psoas and hip rotators are often problem shortened muscle groups. Soft tissue work around the back extensors is often helpful, again maintaining neutral.

Figure 24. Therapist Notes for Posterior Approach Fusion Surgeries

posterior lumbar interbody fusion (PLIF), posterior lateral fusion with or without pedicle screws, combination PLIF/PLF, or "360" fusion. Notes are supplementary to postsurgical fusion therapy protocol.

1. The purpose of this surgery is usually to replace painful degenerated or internally disrupted discs. The surgery can also be done to repair a ruptured disc if the rupture is extensive or if instability is present. The cage implants afford more stability than most fusion devices because they take up most of the intervertebral space and do so with an expansion force into the space. Posterior fusions sometimes have additional hardware. The rehabilitation concepts can also apply to posterior lateral lumbar fusions without interbody fusion, but progression with movement and loading usually must be done more slowly.

2. It is very important to know which levels were fused, and this information should arrive on the therapy prescription. The cage implants are perforated titanium cages that go in the disc space and

are packed with bone shavings. The vertebral bone should then grow through the cage to secure the fusion. The cages generally will increase the intervertebral space at that level and are more secure than bone plugs, but also, they may create a constant stretch on previously lax ligaments and tendons. It is important to know if allograft or autograft fusion was done, as donor site symptoms are common, along with occasional weakness in adjacent muscles which might share attachments or nerve irritation.

3. If the patient is having less pain following the surgery, early therapy is very helpful. Isometric trunk work with the therapist monitoring control of the muscles is a first step. Basic stabilization must be reviewed as the mechanics of neutral spine change a lot following the surgery. The fusion may create the impression that the patient can stabilize their spine easily, so it is important to watch and palpate for muscular control. Abdominals and back extensors both are difficult muscles to recruit, and should be an area of emphasis in every program. Patients will strongly favor proximal extremity muscle groups instead. Oblique abdominals can often be recruited first, but need to be done with minimal trunk motion. Back extensors often come in best by facilitation from the upper body: neck or thoracic spine extension, or by working latissimus and trapezius.

4. Measure and monitor posture, as posterior approach surgeries often tend to have a decreasing lordosis, and completely inactive back extensors. If you notice a changing posture and especially if it is accompanied by increasing backache, a lumbosacral brace may help. Depending on the size of the patient you may opt for semirigid or simple elastic brace. In some cases even a rigid TLSO is appropriate, but only if you have consulted the physician.

5. Often extension-biased aerobic exercise such as the treadmill is best for these patients. Neutral position may need to be strictly maintained for some, and then either arm ergometry or a pool

program can help. If patients can walk without increasing back or leg pain, walking is okay. The pool is great if you have it, but monitor the patient's heart rate to be sure the exercise is aerobic. We believe a good aerobic progression can help patients achieve better early pain control and also minimize weight gain. Low aerobic levels also cause the patients to fatigue before they can benefit from other conditioning attempts, so endurance and aerobic level must be addressed as early as possible.

6. Manual therapy can often help facilitate exercise progression. This is our theory based on our observations of these patients so far. Assisted hip stretching and thoracic spine mobilization with strict attention to maintaining neutral lumbar spine is often helpful. Psoas and hip rotators are often problem shortened muscle groups. Soft tissue work around the back extensors is often helpful, again maintaining neutral. Manual techniques can also be used to help with muscle recruitment in the back extensor area.

Chapter Eight

·,,•●•,,,,,•'••

Managing the Patient following Lumbar Intradiscal Electrothermal Therapy (IDET)

The role of rehabilitation with IDET has not yet been established. This procedure was developed as a less invasive treatment of a degenerative disc. In this procedure, a small catheter heating device is inserted into the disc and the annular wall is heated until the collagen is believed to be reformed. The theory is that the disc wall can be strengthened and repaired with this procedure, and that some of the pain fibers in the annular wall will be ablated. A stress-free postprocedural time is felt to be critical for proper healing of the intervertebral disc, and thus it is suggested that the patient avoid movement of the back for six to twelve weeks (Oratec 1999).

Physical therapy is not recommended until six to twelve weeks postprocedure, and so this protocol has been written with attention to this precaution. As we learn more about the outcomes for these patients, we will be able to tailor the protocol more specifically to their needs. Since this is a new procedure, some of the protocol has been designed to help the physicians who perform the IDET evaluate their outcomes.

One of the companies who manufactures IDET equipment provides a physical therapy protocol (Oratec 1999). This protocol includes many spine stabilization exercises and tests. Six to twelve weeks of inactivity is specified in the Oratec protocol also. Is was the opinion of our group that the progression of the exercises diverged from our approach to spinal rehabilitation. At the request of one of our physicians we developed a protocol (Figure 25) which contains many of the same elements, but begins muscular work earlier and progresses much more slowly.

PRE-IDET EVALUATION

The physical therapy evaluation provides a baseline for outcome measures postprocedure. Evaluation items include similar parameters to those used for many surgical studies:

1. brief gait description;

2. functional mobility screen (timed up and go from sitting and also from supine and picking up an object from the floor);

3. posture measures, sagittal plane, and descriptions of right/left deviations;

4. range of motion of spine and hips;

5. neurologic screen (straight leg raise, lower extremity reflexes, sensory and motor testing);

6. pain drawing; and

7. pre-IDET screen, including Waddell Signs, Oswestry Low Back Pain Questionnaire small checklist of risk factors for chronic pain.

The above evaluation can be done in twenty to thirty minutes, in a checklist format, in order to produce a quick summary for physicians. At the time of the evaluation, there is also an educational opportunity to begin involving the patient in the important recovery process. This can be most easily done if the patient learns basics about the spine, the importance of body mechanics and attention to spine position. Basic information about the IDET procedure can be given at this time. The use of ice for pain, fitting and wearing of brace can also be covered. Bracing is required by most IDET protocols (Oratec).

We would also strongly recommend an attempt to teach muscular bracing exercises for the low back maintaining a neutral spine position. Introducing the muscular system and its importance in the overall health and function of the spine can insure the patient is aware that exercise will be necessary to the recovery process.

Education can be provided in video form, followed by one-on-one time for questions and answers. With a new procedure and careful attention to patient selection and follow-up, the whole package may be accepted by insurance providers, reducing the payer/provider interface to one step.

A primary goal of our protocol is to have the patient ready to reach Maximum Medical Improvement (MMI) in four months, at the most. With careful monitoring and early education, we would work on decreasing that during the time frame of the IDET.

POST-IDET REHABILITATION SCHEDULE

1. FOUR-WEEK EVALUATION

Again, we have a departure from the Oratec protocol (1999) in that we recommend a four week postprocedure physical therapy evaluation. The strategy for this four week evaluation is twofold: 1) to troubleshoot and give the patient two weeks (until the physician's office visit) to work on corrective measures, and 2) to begin spine stabilization muscle recruitment with no lumbar movement. The physician sees the patient for the first time at six weeks and problems can be more accurately identified with the two-week history. When the patients are first seen both by physician and therapist at six weeks, interventions for problems must be determined in a one-time visit. Then there can be a four to six week delay if the patient fails to respond to the intervention. Once again, if stabilization is begun early, it is critical to start the patient on a program of stabilization muscle recruitment and minimize neural tension with no spinal movement. Since it is felt the optimal recovery of the disc following the IDET will occur with a period of immobilization, the patient should be able to demonstrate his or her capability to do basic stabilization muscular control at the six-week checkup.

At the four-week evaluation, problematic patients can be identified, and patients who continue to have symptoms, but will follow recommendations, can receive extra attention. Those who are uncooperative or resistant to the follow-up procedure can be identified and perhaps involved with behavioral medicine. The patients can then have the most appropriate therapy programs prescribed for them.

2. SIX-WEEK POSTPROCEDURE REHABILITATION

Rehabilitation begins, again with a stabilization emphasis and spinal movements only in midranges. The patient continues to exercise in limited trunk range until they can pass Level I spine stabilization screen and have at least an average MET level so that they will not fail muscular support from fatigue alone.

The rehabilitation program will last from four to six weeks until the patient can pass a Level I or II PCT, as described in Chapter 3, and show at least fifty percent reduction in pain. Industrial patients can be transitioned into work hardening any time they are able to pass a Level I PCT, and report a pain level showing fifty percent or more improvement. The average industrial patient could potentially have four to six weeks work hardening to complete the program.

Rehabilitation is completed at ten to twelve weeks post-IDET including four to six weeks therapy on a two to three times per week basis for nonindustrial patients. For industrial patients, rehabilitation is completed at twelve to sixteen weeks post-IDET which includes six to twelve weeks of therapy and then work hardening.

Figure 25. IDET Rehabilitation Protocol

REHABILITATION GOALS, 0-1 week (Note: all time intervals refer to time post-IDET procedure.)

1. Protect spine and treated structures.

2. Maintain strength and endurance in lower extremities (via walking only).

3. Help control pain with heat or cold and attention to spinal position.

REHABILITATION PROGRAM, 0-1 week

1. Instruct patients to avoid all bending, stooping, and twisting. Observe body mechanics as instructed in preprocedure sessions.

2. Limit lifting to ten pounds, occasionally.

3. Remind patients to use brace as ordered by physician.

4. Instruct patient to follow walking program twice a day to pain tolerance and to start recording time of each walk on a daily basis.

5. Remind patients not to drive for amount of time specified by physician (usually two to seven days).

REHABILITATION GOALS, 1-4 weeks (or until postprocedure physical therapy evaluation)

1. Continue protection of spine and treated structures with proper body mechanics and precautions as listed above.

2. Improve strength and endurance in lower extremities (walking only).

3. Start recruitment of spine stabilization muscles, maintaining neutral spine, as instructed preprocedure.

4. Reinforce all Pre-IDET instruction, via telephone interview with patient.

REHABILITATION PROGRAM, 1-4 weeks (We recommend using a video reviewing body mechanics and instructions for these exercises.)

1. Maintain abdominal bracing in corset in full neutral position.

2. Do abdominal bracing with arm reach.

3. Do ankle pumps.

4. Do quad sets, hamstring sets.

5. Practice seated knee extension, with strict attention to neutral spine, and limiting range to that which can be done without radiating pain.

6. Gradually increase walking distance with a goal of one to two miles per day by postprocedure physical therapy evaluation (distance may be divided into morning and evening walks).

7. Continue to wear corset and observe movement limitations:

   a. No bending, stooping, or twisting.

   b. No lifting more than ten pounds until P.T. evaluation.

REHABILITATION GOALS, 4-6 WEEKS

1. Complete physical therapy evaluation of patient. (Use Lumbar Postsurgical Evaluation Form, with no lumbar range of motion measures yet.)

2. Increase endurance and stabilization strength.

3. Begin Level I spine stabilization exercises, based on evaluation findings.

4. Review abdominal bracing and isometrics from the first four weeks postprocedure, if patient is unable to demonstrate.

5. Reassess patient's knowledge of body mechanics and precautions.

REHABILITATION PROGRAM, 4-6 WEEKS.

1. Carry out physical therapy evaluation (using Lumbar Postsurgical Evaluation Form, Chapter 2, Figure 8.)

2. Instruct patient to continue home walking program.

3. Address Level I spine stabilization, assigning core exercises plus any needed to address positive findings on the P.T. evaluation.

4. Carry out abdominal bracing assessment and reinstruction, if necessary.

5. Perform functional screen for proper body mechanics, to include:

a. lifting five pounds from floor;

b. moving from supine to sitting to supine; and

c. performing a timed "up and go" test.

6. Instruct patient to record exercises and walking daily on flow sheet.

REHABILITATION GOALS, 6-12 WEEKS

1. Continue emphasis on attention to proper posture and body mechanics, with good support of the spine.

2. Progress strength, endurance, and flexibility to maximize functional activity.

REHABILITATION PROGRAM, 6-12 WEEKS.

1. Start formal physical therapy two to three times per week.

2. Select treatment interventions based on each positive evaluation finding. (Refer to postsurgical evaluation findings and suggested therapy intervention list in Chapter 10, Figure 27. Suggestions for the IDET procedure itself can be found in Figures 28 and 29.)

3. Help patients with minimal to no limitations learn Level I stabilization and reconditioning in preparation for passing Level I PCT.

a. Practice basic stabilization, especially of the PCT test exercises once patient can demonstrate good control of neutral spine.

b. Use endurance work to prepare for first treadmill MET level estimation at about eight weeks.

c. Increase lifting limit once patient is able to pass Level I PCT; no more than twenty-five percent of their grip strength per week.

4. Patients with several identified problems focus first on pain relief and introduction of stabilization muscle recruitment with attention to least painful positions and movements.

5. Progress industrial patients to work hardening.

Figure 26. Patient Instructions

After IDET (Intradiscal Electrothermal Therapy)

1. No lifting over ten pounds until your six week postprocedure follow-up, unless your physician tells you otherwise.

2. No bending, no stooping, and no twisting for the first six weeks. Activities and movements should not be painful. Walk as much as possible, several times a day for short distances at first. Wear your brace as instructed by your physician. In most cases, the brace should be worn as much as possible.

3. Use good body mechanics when changing positions. When getting up from lying down, always log roll to your side *first*. Then sit up by pushing up from your side.

4. Support the low back with a pillow whenever you sit. Avoid prolonged sitting. Thirty minutes should be the maximum amount of time seated.

5. Preferred sleeping positions: on your side with knees bent and a pillow between, or on your back with pillows under your knees. Some patients obtain relief from wearing a brace at night, loosened slightly.

6. Driving may not be allowed for the first two to seven days post-procedure.

7. Return to work release *must* be given by your physician before you return to work.

8. It is best to avoid sex the first two weeks, or if pain increases significantly after the procedure. Once you resume sex, you still must observe the lifting and bending restrictions listed above and wear your brace. Sidelying is the safest approach.

9. In order to help you move more easily when you first get up from lying down, try the following. Turn on to your back, bend your knees as much as possible comfortably with both feet flat on the bed. Then, *gently,* rock your knees from side to side only moving about an inch in each direction at a pace of about two per second. Try to do this for two to three minutes. It will help circulation and be a warm-up which will allow you to move more easily afterward. Rocking in a rocking chair can help in the same way. Always rock *gently.*

Please call the physical therapy department if you have any questions.

Chapter Nine

..••●●●•••••••••

Managing Patients
following Selected Lumbar Injections

EPIDURAL STEROID INJECTIONS (ESI)

ESIs for the lumbar spine are often given as a first line of defense for lumbar syndromes where disc pathology is suspected, especially if radiating leg pain is present (Cyriax 1980; Sullivan 1992). If the ESI is successful and the desired effect of pain relief occurs, it is an excellent opportunity for rehabilitation to take place. The rehabilitation can be designed to augment the effects of the injection.

The first stage of rehabilitation is the reinforcement of disc protection via posture, positioning, and support. Identification of neutral spine positions where symptoms are minimal to absent and then recruiting trunk muscle support for these positions is key. This portion of the management is similar to that for any patient with lumbar disc problems (Donelson et al. 1990; Saal and Saal 1989). Also, many practitioners feel that early work on neural mobility is important. This emphasizes mobility along the nerve pathway, minimizing areas of unnecessary tension (Kornberg and McCarthy

1992). For example, tightness in hamstrings, hip rotators, or calves can each limit the excursion of the sciatic nerve, as well as its blood supply, and therefore, could compromise optimal nerve function.

Once the symptoms are under control following ESI, correcting pathomechanics which may accompany the original problem is important. Common pathomechanics include:

1. asymmetrical posture or *lateral shift* in McKenzie's terms (1991);

2. decreased muscle recruitment capability; and/or

3. abnormal lumbar mobility.

Postural correction may still be needed after the symptoms have resolved, as in time continued deviated posture can result in repeated pain patterns. Muscle recruitment has been shown to be altered in key back extensor groups with many lumbar spine pathologies (Hides et al. 1996). Also proprioception has been shown to be decreased with chronic low back pain, which can in turn diminish muscle recruitment capabilities (Gill and Callaghan 1998). Therefore, muscle reeducation, in particular for the trunk muscles, is an important component for rehabilitation so that optimal function can be restored.

General spine conditioning can benefit patients undergoing ESIs just as it does other conservative care spine patients. It can help the patient safely resume full activity, once they have completed the first stage of spine care. The nonsurgical protocol in Chapter 1 applies to these patients, after the initial focus on the steps taken to follow-up on the intent of the injection, which is pain control. Suggested post-ESI exercises are found in Chapter 10, Figures 28 and 29.

ZYGAPOPHYSIAL JOINT INJECTIONS (Z-Joint Injections)

These injections are done diagnostically to identify pain-generating z-joints (also termed *facets*). The injections can also treat the pain, once the offending joints are identified. Z-joint injections are intended to be used as an adjunct to aggressive, conservative spine care (Dreyfuss et al. 1994). Although the best specific conservative care has yet to be identified for this patient population, both manipulation and carefully selected exercise are felt to be among the most effective choices. Painful joints are likely to be related to faulty mechanics which either caused or were caused by the pain. With the pain eliminated, the environment is ideal for restoring normal joint function.

We have had the good fortune of developing rehabilitation protocols for studies with Dreyfuss and his colleagues, spine specialists who have been investigating and publishing studies on various aspects of spinal injections and conservative care for several years (Dreyer et al. 1994, Dreyfuss et al. 1995). One proposed study was designed to look at combined effects of injections, manipulation, and active rehabilitation on patients with diagnosed z-joint pathology. The basic z-joint protocol involves a careful postural and spinal mobility evaluation to identify possible mechanical factors contributing to the z-joint dysfunction. For example, an excessive lordosis can add unnecessary compression to z-joints (Dreyer et al. 1994). Any postural right/left asymmetry can add load to the z-joints on one side of the spine as well.

Muscle imbalances can further increase mechanical problems. The common *cross weakness* pattern, with tight hip flexors and lumbar extensors, and weak abdominals and hip extensors, tends to reinforce an excessive lordosis and add muscular force to the already increased load on the z-joints. The z-joints are not designed for sustained load (Dreyer et al. 1994). Identifying all of these factors in a careful evaluation and addressing each factor with a corrective force, via manipulation and/or muscle contraction, can help restore normal function to the z-joints. The principles of matching active exercise to evaluation findings is discussed in detail in the next chapter. Manual therapy and manipulation can also help maximize joint function, but is not within the scope of this text. There are several texts which describe manual therapy and manipulation of the lumbar spine for z-joint problems (Basmajian and Nyberg 1993; Cyriax 1980; Greenman 1996) It is important to note that based on our experience, we recommend initiating therapy for these patients immediately after the injections.

Once again, following the initial pain management stage, and once fairly normal range of motion is established in the lumbar spine, the rest of the nonsurgical protocol described in Chapter 1 can be used to complete the program. Some specific suggestions for exercises for patients following z-joint injections are found in Chapter 10, Figures 28 and 29.

Chapter Ten

••••●●●•••••••

Exercise Selection for Spine Patients

There has been a fervent search over the years for The Best Spine Exercise. We have seen heated debate over various forms of spine exercise, and passionate arguments over which muscle groups are most important to spinal function. For a long time therapists could be split into camps which believed in the benefits of spinal flexion or extension. This has all been heightened by equipment manufacturers attempting to come up with a device with which one can get the most improvement with the least amount of effort.

As many therapists will agree, in truth there are many effective exercise programs available, and many options for helping spine function with exercise. Much of the success of any exercise regimen is determined by the amount of enthusiastic regular exercise done by the participant. Also important, however, is the specificity of the exercise to the patient's body type, experience with exercise, motor learning capabilities, and existing mechanical dysfunction. The *existing mechanical dysfunction* includes both that which has occurred because of the spine pathology/surgery, and any pre-existing suboptimal musculoskeletal functions. These factors add up to a lot of variables! It only makes sense that a single program that can address all of the variables probably doesn't exist.

This chapter will present some exercise concepts, with several exercise references which can be helpful in selecting a "best exercise program" for a patient with spinal dysfunction. In prior chapters, reference is made to specific exercises which we have selected for our protocols. By understanding our rationale in the selection process, readers may formulate their own ideas on exercise selection priorities for a specific case load. No one has come up with the perfect program yet.

Often, there is a necessary amount of trial and error in exercise program design. It is difficult to predict all of an individual's possible responses to exercise, and therefore errors are often made when designing programs for patients. An unfortunate tendency is for the patient to go back to the physician after a poor response to exercise. Many times, both physician and patient will conclude that a single poor response to some exercise is an indication that all exercise is useless and may hurt the patient. Thus, it is paramount for therapists to make strong efforts to educate physicians about exercise. With patients, it can help to explain *before* beginning the program that exercise is like medicine. Not all of it works the same for all people, and sometimes the only way to find the right exercise is through trial and error. Making the analogy of not giving up on all medicine if one doesn't work helps many patients.

In this chapter, attention will be placed on two areas. The first and most in-depth part will cover exercise selection concepts, based on two main areas: 1) evaluation findings showing musculoskeletal and functional deficits in the individual patient; and 2) musculoskeletal factors which may help augment the effects of the surgery. The second section of the chapter will deal with exercise progression and attention to factors such as frequency, intensity, and duration, as well as strategies to overcome plateaus.

EXERCISE SELECTION CONCEPTS

Once again, it was our good fortune to have participated in some clinical trials with local physicians. Physical therapy was usually not a variable in the studies, but was included in some of the patient management. It was necessary, therefore, to come up with a single system of exercise selection that could be individualized for the patient, but in a consistent manner. We chose to do this by matching exercises with evaluation findings. For example, if a subject had forward head carriage on evaluation, we included a postural retraining exercise in their program. We did have a group of *core exercises* designed to augment the procedures involved in the studies; lumbar facet injections and lumbar epidural steroid injections. The benefit of this work for us is that we saw the value in giving rationale for every choice we made in the patient's care. We realized that we should use this level of care for all of our patients. This allows us to backtrack and more accurately identify sources of problems when they occur. It also allows us to improve and maintain our consistency from therapist to therapist in our management. It makes program improvement much more objective.

The evaluation form in Chapter 2 (Figure 8) has some small check boxes in the left hand margin by each category heading. These have been placed on the form so the therapist can check a box if the patient has an abnormal finding which could be addressed by therapy in that category. The therapist can use the checked boxes to formulate a problem list at the end of the evaluation and then be *certain* to address each problem with a component of the therapy program. If a problem list has redundant findings, this suggests extra emphasis on intervention in that area.

Some broad categories of problems and example interventions are listed below:

Problem	Intervention
radiating leg pain	neural mobilization via specific active and assisted (manual therapy) movements; modalities to facilitate movements and help with pain control, if needed
excessive lordosis	stretching lumbodorsal fascia, abdominal strengthening, upright postural retraining, hip flexor stretching
weak hip or back extensors	strengthening first in positions of maximal recruitment, then in functional tasks
hip rotator tightness/ weakness or right/left imbalance	hip rotator stretching/ strengthening manual therapy for facilitation

More detail, with examples of specific exercises presented later in this chapter, is given in Figure 27. In this table, we are suggesting exercises that we feel may help correct a given problem identified on evaluation. Not all possibilities for exercise selection or all of the possible evaluation findings are included in this table, but it should provide enough examples to give a therapist a picture of our rationale.

The second area of exercise selection deals with the specific surgery. When surgery alters architecture in any way, invades muscle integrity, or has the potential of creating scar interference with smooth functional movements, there are opportunities for therapy to significantly help the patient. Again, important areas of emphasis are outlined in the previous chapters which covered the different types of surgeries and procedures. To review some of the ideas from the previous chapters, examples are listed below:

Surgery	Intervention Concept
Decompression lumbar laminectomy (for stenosis, Chapter 6)	trunk strengthening, usually with flexion bias; also lumbar flexion mobility and hip flexibility for neural mobilization
Laminectomy for HNP (Chapter 6)	usually helped by back extensor recruitment and stabilization work reinforcing support of spine during activity
Lumbar interbody fusion (Chapter 7)	may be sensitive to upright at first, may be helped with initial non-weightbearing exercise; emphasis is on creating muscular support for the spine with stabilization; thoracic mobility often helps these patients; work on donor site if autograft bone used (hip stretches)
IDET (Chapter 8)	treated initially more as a fusion patient in order to protect the disc; mobility often must be restricted completely the first several weeks

For more detail regarding exercise selection for specific surgeries, two tables are included in Figure 28 and 29. In these tables, several surgeries and specific exercises are suggested. Critical attention must be paid to symptoms produced during various movements,

Suggested Exercise	Evaluation Finding											
	xkyph	xlord	lat shift	limit L flex	limit L ext	SLR+	PKF+	funct+	sens flex	sens ext	sens wt	FHFSh
Fig. 30 Recruit abs w/ back support		X		X						X		
Fig. 31 Basic recruitment of back ex			X		X				X			
Fig. 32 Back ext recruit w/ spine support	X								X			
Fig. 33 Funct. Act. stand w/ neutral spine								X				
Fig. 34 Neural Mobl. sciatic nerve						X				X	X	
Fig. 35 Hip flexor and Quad stretches							X		X			
Fig. 36 Thoracic/Ribcage mobility work	X											
Fig. 37 Lower abdominal work		X		X						X		
Fig. 38 Self mobl. techq for L & T spine	X	X										X
Low Back I				#1-5					X	#5-8		
Low Back II				#6-9								
Low Back III	←			Progression to Level II								→
Supported Low Back									X		X	
Instructions for controlling leg pain			X								X	
Seated trunk circles												X
Ribcage				X	X						#6	
Cervical Range of Motion				X	X							X
Upper Extremity Theraband												X
Anterior Tib (Ankle Pumping)						X		X			X	

Figure 27. Table of Suggested Exercise Selections
for Specific Evaluation Findings

Key for Figure 27

Refer to the evaluation techniques described in Chapter 2. For each of the following common findings listed below, we have indicated some exercise selections we would choose. An *x* indicates that all pictures in a given figure or exercise instruction sheet (found in this chapter) are applicable. Specific numbers are listed if we would limit the choices within a selection.

Evaluation findings:

xkyph	excessive kyphosis
xlord	excessive lordosis
lat shift	lateral shift
limit L flex	limited lumbar flexion
limit L ext	limited lumbar extension
SLR+	positive straight leg raise
PKF+	positive femoral nerve stretch
sens flex	position sensitivity to flexion (see Chapter 1)
funct+	unable to pass functional screens
sens ext	position sensitivity to extension
sens wt	weight-bearing sensitivity
FHFSh	forward head, forward shoulders (posture section)

and exercises may need to be modified considerably for different individuals. As always, any increase in radiating pain with a movement is a relative contraindication for that movement at the time. In Figure 28, exercises that can usually be done within the first few weeks of therapy evaluation are indicated. In Figure 29, suggestions are made for exercise progression, once the patient is experienced with more basic movements. As a rule of thumb, the exercise progressions in Figure 29 are more appropriate after a patient can pass a Level I PCT.

It is often helpful to consider the effects of the surgery tissue by tissue, so that all musculoskeletal components that can maximize recovery are included (McFarland 1994). Some ideas on this concept are presented in Chapter 11.

EXERCISE PROGRESSION

This is a challenging area for the therapist, as precise progression is critical to the most rapid result of the exercise. Unfortunately, in the present health care environment, the evaluating therapist often is not the person supervising the exercise, and progression may suffer as a result. However, with clear guidelines and tracking of the exercise, progression can be built into the program.

Importance of attention to frequency, intensity, and duration have been well-researched, although some specifics regarding these are still disputed (ACSM 1995). It is agreed that progression needs to be made in at least one of the three areas to produce continuing change. Arriving at the best numbers for the spine patient has been an ongoing challenge, and will be helped by more therapists reporting specifics of their programs. Therefore, documenting how many times per week, how many repetitions of which exercises and how the intensity was increased for a given population of patients could help better define rehabilitation for our patients. Unfortunately, with large numbers of diverse patients, this is difficult to do.

For many therapy programs, however, especially in the era of the home program, including any method of progression at all will be an improvement. It is extremely important, of course, that the patient understands the idea behind progression. Very often, with a good understanding, the patient can be the best producer of a productive program. It helps if the patient understands that on a day when they don't feel like increasing intensity, if they increase duration, progress can still be made. The idea of alternating intensive activity, and longer duration low-level exercise can be very helpful lifelong advice. Patients may sustain their interest in exercise on a more long-term basis if it is varied.

EXERCISE ILLUSTRATIONS

On the following pages, illustrations of exercises are grouped by exercise type. Most are familiar exercises for therapists, but the instruction and attention to precision movements is the key to success with them. Some of that instruction should be verbal and with guided demonstration for the patient, to be sure the movement is achieving the desired goal. These illustrations should serve the therapist in suggesting various strategies to work on typical problem areas for spine patients.

Stabilization work has many possible approaches, and will likely be the most successful if there is some concentrated practice in muscle recruitment, particularly of abdominals (Figures 30 and 37) and back extensors (Figures 31 and 32), in varying positions. The new book on segmental stabilization of the spine (Richardson et al. 1999) is an excellent resource for expanding on a stabilization program as well as improving precision of exercise.

Suggested Ex Selection	Lumbar Procedure							
	LLH	SDLL	ALIF	PLF/I	360	IDET	ESI	ZJI
Fig.30 Recruit abdominal w/ back support		X	X				X	X
Fig. 31 Basic recruitment of back ex	X			#1-3	#1-3	#1-3	#2,3	
Fig.32 Back ext recruit w/ spine support	X			#1		X	X	
Fig. 33 Funct. activity stand w/ neutral spine	X	X	#2-4	#2-4	#2-4	X		X
Fig.34 Neural Mobl. sciatic nerve	X	X	X	#1	X	X	X	X
Fig. 35 Hip flexor and Quad stretches	X	X	#4	#4	#4		X	
Fig.36 Thoracic/Ribcage mobility work	#1-3	#1-3	#1-3	#1-3	#1-3	#1-3	#1-3	#1-3
Fig. 37 Lower abdominal work		X						X
Fig. 38 Self mobl. techniques for L & T spine							#1	X
Low Back I	#1-5	#5-8	#5-8	#1-3,5	#1-3,5	#1-3,5	#1-5	#5-8
Low Back II	#1-5,8	#6-9	#6-9					#6-9
Low Back III								X
Supported Low Back	X	X	X	X	X	X	X	X
Instructions for controlling leg pain	X	X					X	
Seated trunk circle								X
Ribcage	#1-5	#1-5	#1-4	#1-4	#1-4	#1-4	#1-6	
Cervical Range of Motion	X	X	X	X	X	X	X	X
Upper Extremity Theraband	X	X	X	X	X	X	X	
Anterior Tib (Calf Pumping)	X	X	X	X	X	X	X	

Figure 28. Table of Suggested Exercise
Selections for Early Rehabilitation
Following Specific Lumbar Procedures

Key for Figure 28

This table indicates common initial exercise choices given to patients within the first few weeks following their postsurgical physical therapy evaluation. Bear in mind that this may be a program given in the first few weeks after surgery, or not until the six week or initial office visit with the surgeon. Usually the surgeon will have a definite preference for time frame.

All exercises must be given with careful education of the patient regarding watching for symptom changes. For example, if an exercise increases radiating pain, the patient must understand to discontinue the exercise until they see the therapist. There are more choices given on the table than would ever be given to a patient at one time. However, combining these choices with those recommended by evaluation findings can help prioritize the selection process. As in Figure 27, an *x* indicates that any of the exercises in a given figure or instruction sheet may be chosen. Numbers indicate a limited choice.

Lumbar Procedures

LLH	lumbar laminectomy, or nonfusion procedure for herniated disc
SDLL	decompression lumbar laminectomy for stenosis
ALIF	anterior lumbar interbody fusion
PLF/I	posterior lateral fusion (PLF) or posterior lumbar interbody fusion (PLIF)
360	any combination of anterior and posterior approach, or PLIF and PLF
IDET	Intradiscal Electrothermal Therapy procedure
ESI	epidural steroid injection
ZJI	zygapophysial (facet) joint injection

Suggested Progression	LLH	SDLL	ALIF	PLF/I	360	IDET	ESI	ZJI
				Lumbar Procedure				
Fig. 30 Recruit abdominal w/ back support	X			X	X	X		
Fig. 31 Basic recruitment of back ex		X	X					X
Fig. 32 Back ext recruit w/ spine support		X	X	#2,3	X			X
Fig. 33 Funct. activity stand w/ neutral spine	C	C	X	X	X	X	C	C
Fig. 34 Neural Mobl. sciatic nerve	C	C	C	C	C	C	X	
Fig. 35 Hip flexor and Quad stretches		X	X		X			
Fig. 36 Thoracic / Ribcage mobility work	ALL	ALL	C	C	C	C	ALL	ALL
Fig. 37 Lower abdominal work	X			X	X	X		
Fig. 38 Self mobl. techniques for L & T spine	X	X			X			
Low Back I			#6-8	#6-8	#6-8			
Low Back II	X	X				X	X	X
Low Back III	X	X	X	X	X		X	X
Supported Low Back								
Instructions for controlling leg pain			X	X	X	X		X
Seated trunk circles			X	X	X	X		
Ribcage	#6-8	#6-8	C	C	C	C	#6-8	#6-8
Cervical Range of Motion								
Upper Extremity Theraband	X	X	X	X	X	X	X	
Anterior Tib (Ankle Pumping)								

Figure 29. Table of Suggested Exercise Selections for
Progression of Rehabilitation Program
Following Specific Lumbar Procedures

Key for Figure 29

This figure indicates choices for progression, usually after the patient has been in active therapy for a few weeks at least. Progressions are most safely done if the patient can pass a Level I PCT first. Several suggestions are made in this table, but there are still many more! The table indicates the ones we use most frequently and again the programs vary greatly between individuals. Symptoms must be watched carefully.

X indicates a new choice or an exercise for progression. *C* indicates one we might continue as a part of the patient's core program. *ALL* indicates that although the exercises were limited to certain ones on a given figure or instruction sheet, progression can include them all. Again specific numbers are given if limitations still apply. These exercises are examples of a first level of progression. Many patients will go beyond this level.

Neural mobilization for the lower extremities can help reduce inhibition due to pain that might interfere with progress in these exercises. The neural mobilization exercises in Figure 34 and 35 also key in on flexibility in important muscle groups, such as the iliopsoas, quads, and hamstrings. Hip rotators are also important, but are addressed in other exercises.

Finally, motor control issues are addressed in exercises for balance, repeated practice of functional activities with attention to body mechanics, and the increasing coordination demands of the stabilization exercise progressions. These progressions have been well described in many therapeutic exercise books, and will not be covered here; however, a few examples of the motor control activities are given in Figures 33, 42, and 44.

In the following exercise illustrations, written as instruction sheets for patients, blank spaces have been left for the therapist to indicate number of repetitions to start. We have found that this can make or break an exercise program for patients who are hesitant in any way. We have not found a formula for ideal number of repetitions, but give our general guideline. We usually start with one set of ten repetitions for younger or more fit patients, and start with five repetitions for older or less fit patients.

Figure 30. Examples of Level I Spine Stabilization

Recruiting Abdominals with Back Fully Supported

1. *Hand knee push.* This is an isometric exercise, where the right hand presses against the right knee in the position shown for a ten second hold. Repeat with the left hand pressing on the left knee. Alternate to complete _____ times on each side. Then press with the opposite hand for another set, to recruit the oblique abdominals.

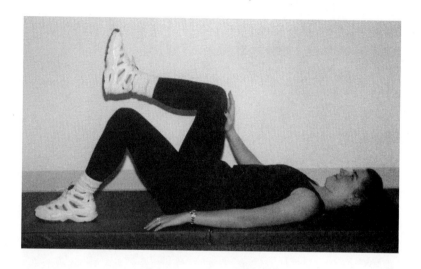

2. *Partial curl up.* Keeping the chin off of the chest and hands behind the head, press the low back into the floor and lift the head up using abdominal muscle contraction. Move with a slow, smooth continuous motion _____ times.

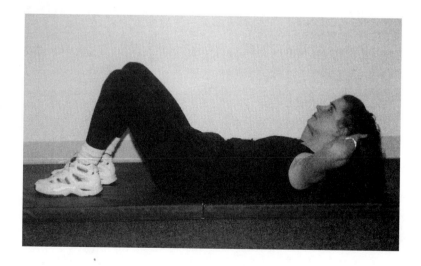

3. *Diagonal curl.* This movement does not involve much rotation. You are directing your right shoulder toward your left knee, in a similar slow controlled motion _____ times. Repeat to the other side.

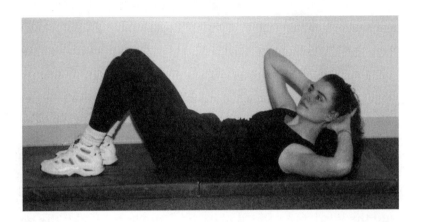

FORM NOTES: If hands are held behind the head, it is important to keep elbows back, as shown in the illustrations. If you have trouble keeping the elbows in this position during the head lift, modify the arm position to either folded across the chest or with hands crossed to opposite shoulders.

Also, if there is neck pain with exercises 2 or 3 in this group, focus on exercise 1 only, and increase the repetitions.

Figure 31. Examples of Level I Spine Stabilization

*Basic Stabilization for Recruitment of Back Extensors
and Co-contraction with Abdominals*

1. *Prone arm and leg lifts.* Lie face down with arms at sides. A pillow may be used under the trunk to minimize arching of the low back. Tighten abdominal muscles to keep the spine still, then

slowly lift one straight arm with the palm of the hand facing the ceiling, then lower it to the floor. Repeat with the other arm. Alternate arms _____ times each. Then lift one straight leg at a time no more than two to three inches off the floor and lower. Repeat with other leg, then alternate _____ times each.

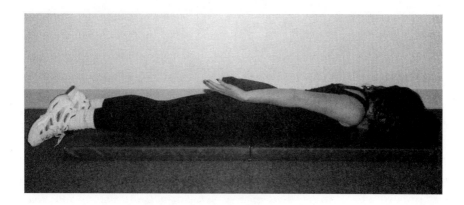

FORM NOTES: If there is back or leg pain with the leg lifts, be sure the abdominal muscles are tight and the low back is not moving at all. If back pain still occurs, try simply bending the knee to a right angle. If this exercise cannot be done without pain, consult the therapist before continuing.

2. *Opposite arm and leg stretch with no movement of the low back.* Lying on your back with knees bent, lift left arm up over your head (as shown) as you slide your right foot away from you, straightening the right leg. Be sure that your back does not arch at all during this movement. Repeat with the other arm and leg for a total of _____ times on each side. If you cannot hold your back still throughout the exercise, try going only part way with your arm and leg.

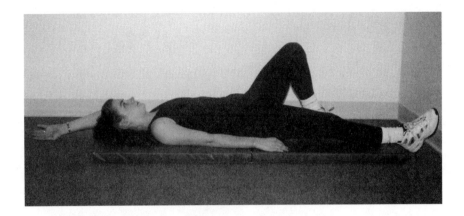

3. *Bridging.* Lying on your back with knees bent. Find the least painful "neutral position" of your low back and tighten the abdominal muscles to maintain this position, then slowly lift the hips off the floor *only as high as you can without moving your low back.* Go up in two counts while breathing out, then lower yourself to the floor in four counts while breathing in. Repeat _____ times.

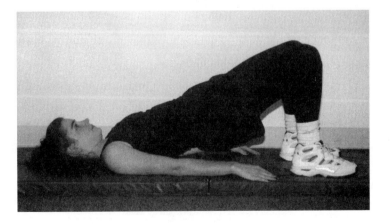

4. *Beginning bird dog.* On the floor on all fours, find the least painful position of your low back and tighten the abdominal muscles to maintain this position. The head should be looking straight at the floor. Breathe out as you lift one leg straight up but no higher than six inches off the floor. Breathe in as you return that leg to starting position. Repeat with the other leg for a total of _____ times on each side.

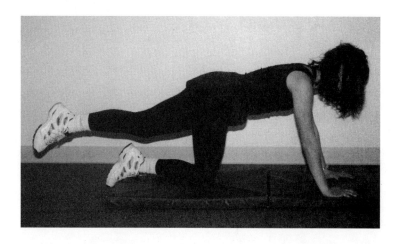

FORM NOTES: If these exercises are painful, you are probably not identifying or holding neutral properly. Discuss this with your therapist. Often small changes in starting position or smaller movements can help.

Figure 32. Examples of Level I Spine Stabilization:

Back Extensor Recruitment with Spine Supported

In all three of these exercises, you start by lying across a chair or foot stool with the trunk supported from chest to hips. If there is too much arch in the low back, a pillow may be added under the abdomen. Before beginning any of these three movements, tighten the stomach muscles and breathe in. Be sure that the head moves as little as possible during these exercises, and look straight down at the floor throughout the movements.

1. *Arm and leg lift over chair.* Lift one leg and opposite arm no higher than parallel to the floor as you slowly breathe out. The other foot stays in contact with the floor and the other hand can hold on to the chair leg, if needed. Lower the leg and arm back to the floor as you breathe in, then repeat with the other arm and leg. Complete _____ lifts with each side.

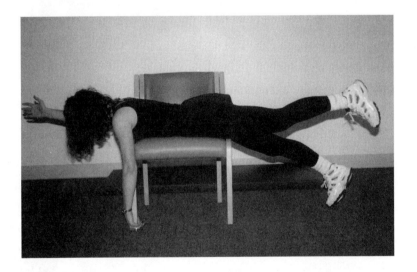

2. *Prone double arm lift over chair.* Keeping both feet on the floor, slowly lift both arms toward the ceiling as you breathe out. Do not bring the arms above the level of your head. Lift up for a two second count, hold for two seconds, then lower for two seconds. Repeat _____ times.

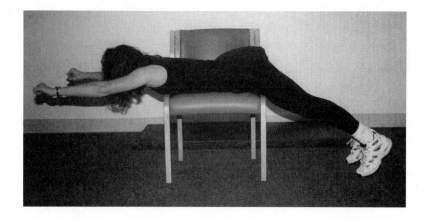

3. *Prone double leg lift over chair.* Hold on to the chair legs or place both hands on the floor. Slowly lift both straight legs up parallel with the floor as you breathe out. Lift in two counts and hold for two counts. Then lower for two counts as you breathe in. Repeat _____ times.

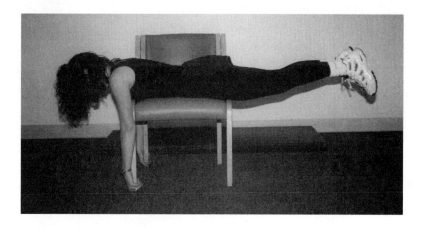

FORM NOTES: Be sure to hold the abdominal muscles tight throughout these movements.

Figure 33. Examples of Practiced Functional Activity Maintaining Neutral Spine

Controlled Standing and Sitting and Balance Practice.

In each of these exercises begin standing with feet slightly apart. Arch your back as much as you can, then flatten your back as much as you can and determine your most comfortable position. This position is called *neutral spine* for standing. Brace your back with neutral spine by tightening your abdominal muscles without changing the position of your back. If you place your hands on the pelvis, you can monitor how well you maintain neutral spine during these exercises. If you have trouble with balance, you can have your hands at your sides.

1. *Straight back forward bend.* Bend the knees slightly then bend forward from the hips, trying not to move the rest of the trunk at all. Bend only as far forward as you can without pain, and no further forward than shown in the illustration. Breathe in as you bend forward and breathe out as you return to standing. Repeat _____ times.

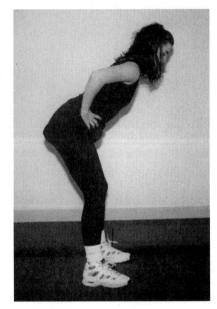

2. *Slow sit downs.* In a standing position with neutral spine as described above, have a chair close behind you, and sit slowly into
the chair over a ten to twenty second time period. You may need
to work up to being able to control this movement over twenty
seconds. As soon as your buttocks touch the chair, return to
standing immediately. Then slowly lower yourself again. Repeat
_____ times. This exercise will help you get up out of most chairs
and even low seats more easily!

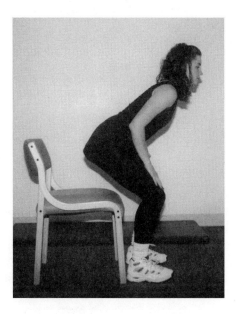

3. *Single leg balance.* After finding your neutral spine and bracing
with your abdominals, see if you can balance on one foot.
Staying on just one foot, shift your weight to the ball and toes
of the foot, then back to the heel still keeping your whole foot
on the floor. It is a slight weight shift. Try alternating the shift
from ball of foot to heel ten times. Then without putting the

other foot down, shift from inside of the foot to outside of the foot, alternately pressing your arch into the floor, then lifting it up ten times. Repeat with the other leg.

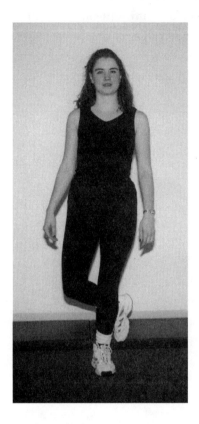

4. *Single leg partial knee bends and hip hike.* If you were able to do all of the weight shifting in Exercise 3 without losing your balance, try doing ten small knee bends on the standing leg (mini single leg squats), and finish by hiking the opposite hip up to the side ten times. Repeat with the other leg.

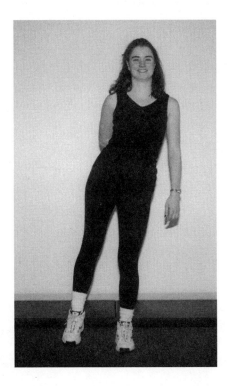

Figure 34. Example Exercises for Neural Mobilization

Sciatic Nerve

It is critical for all of these exercises that a gentle pull is felt, but no pain. If radiating leg pain is severe, it may be necessary to work on ankle and knee mobility first, and then progress to stretches involving the hip.

1. *Progressive straight leg raise, part one.* Lying on your back with knees bent, lift one leg with knee bent toward the chest. Hold the thigh

in toward the chest, but not in close enough to pull on the hip. With the thigh remaining stationary, slowly lift and lower the foot to the point where a pull is felt behind the knee, but *no pain*. Lift and lower the foot slowly ten times holding the stretch a few seconds at the top each time. Repeat with the other leg.

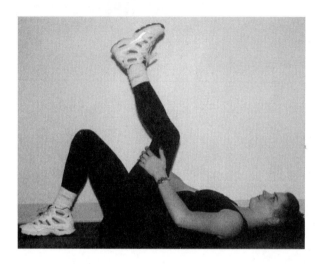

2. *Progressive straight leg raise, part two.* Return to starting position (with knees bent), then lift one bent leg toward the chest, and slowly straighten the knee as much as possible, as in part one. In this exercise, hold the foot up as high as possible, then flex and point the foot. Note that the knee should not fully extend. If the knee can extend fully, try pulling the thigh in closer to the chest where knee extension is not possible. It is not uncommon to feel some tingling in the toes during this movement, but it should not be painful.

3. *Wall stretch with tension on one leg.* Use a wall to support a straight leg raise to the level you can comfortably keep one knee straight and leave it in this position for two to three minutes. Try some

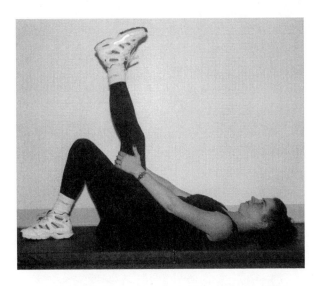

gentle ankle movement while in this position, and this should increase the stretch, but not be painful. If large ankle movements are painful, try a smaller movement, or even just moving the toes.

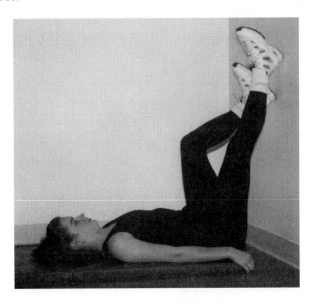

4. *Wall stretch with tension on both legs.* For some individuals, it is easier to do Exercise 3 with both legs at the same time. Try it!

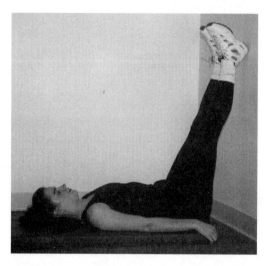

5. *Seated straight leg stretch.* Begin sitting upright and fully straighten one leg in front of you. Try pointing and flexing the foot of the

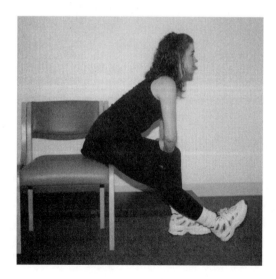

straight leg leaving the heel on the floor. If you do not feel a stretch with this movement, try bending forward at the hips only, keeping your back straight. Place your hands on the bent leg that you are not stretching to support the upper body.

Figure 35. Example Exercises for Hip Flexor and Quadriceps Stretch

with Neural Mobilization for the Femoral Nerve

1. *Kneeling hip flexor stretch.* Kneeling on one knee as shown, tighten the abdominal muscles and tuck both hips under you, which should flatten the lower back. If you are doing this stretch properly, you will feel the stretch in the front of the hip of the kneeling leg. Hold each stretch for twenty to thirty seconds. Repeat three times on each leg.

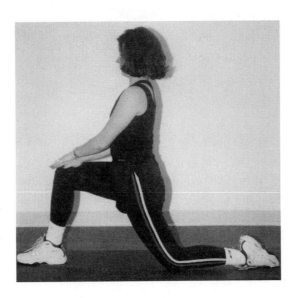

2. *Standing hip flexor stretch.* Stand about two feet in front of a chair or bench. Place one foot on the chair (as shown). Keeping your back straight, lean toward the chair, pressing hips forward first. Tighten your abdominal muscles and do not let your back arch. This stretch should be felt in the front of the hip and thigh of the standing leg. Hold for twenty to thirty seconds, and repeat three times on each leg.

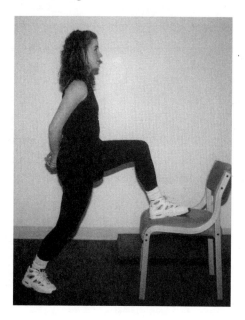

3. *Standing quad and hip flexor stretch.* Facing away from a chair or bench, place the top of your foot on the seat (as shown). The bent knee should be off the front of the seat. Bend the knee of the standing leg slightly, flatten the low back by tightening the abdominal muscles and pulling the hips forward. The stretch should be felt in the front of the thigh of the leg that is on the chair. Hold twenty to thirty seconds for each stretch. Repeat three times on each leg.

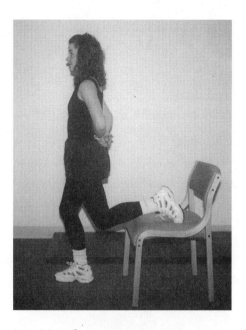

4. *Sidelying quad and hip flexor stretch.* Lying on your side with knees bent slightly to the front, grasp the ankle of the top leg with your hand and pull your foot slowly toward the buttock. Hold at a point where a mild stretch is felt in the front of the thigh, then tighten the abdominal muscles and flatten the lower back. This should increase the stretch in the front of the hip and thigh of the top leg. Hold twenty to thirty seconds, then turn on the other side for the other leg. Repeat three times on each leg.

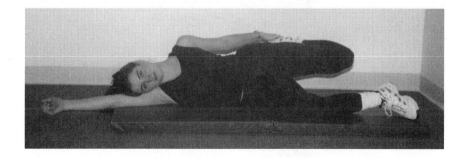

Figure 36. Examples of Stretching for Thoracic Mobility

to Facilitate Better Lumbar and Cervical Control

The first three exercises can be done sitting or standing.

1. *Ribcage stretch overhead.* Grasping both hands overhead, stretch one arm up at a time opening the ribcage on that side. The movement should be slow, with a pause when the arm reaches as high as it can go. Alternate arms _____times on each side.

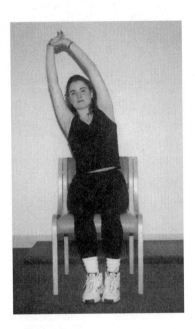

2. *Ribcage stretch for front of chest.* Grasp your hands behind you, being sure to keep your back straight, and avoid tipping your head back. Lift the grasped hands up as high as possible, stretching the fronts of the shoulders. Use a slow movement with a pause at the top. Repeat _____ times.

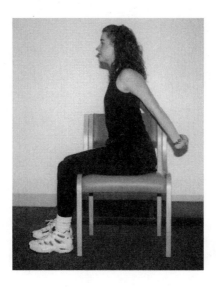

3. *Ribcage stretch for back of chest.* Grasp your hands in front of you and press them forward as you drop your head and round your back slightly. You should feel the stretch in the upper back between the shoulder blades. Repeat _____ times.

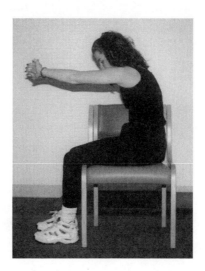

4a. *Camel and cat.* On all fours, first let your back sag toward the floor as you lift your head.

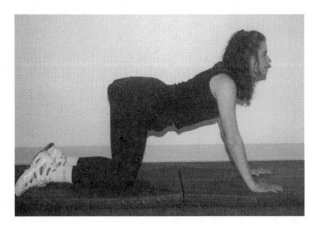

4b. Then drop your head down and pull your stomach up toward the ceiling, rounding your back as high as possible. The arms should not bend at all during either of these movements. Movements should be slow with a pause at both the end of the upward movement and the end of the downward movement.

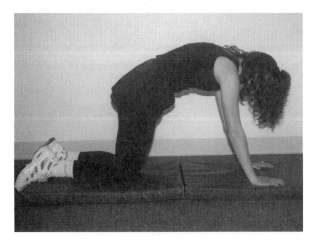

Figure 37. Recruiting Abdominals
with Lower Abdominal Emphasis

1. *Supported dead bugs.* Lying on your back with feet propped on a low stool or step bench, identify neutral spine and brace with the abdominals. Lift one foot a few inches off the bench, then bring the other up next to it; then lower the first foot back to the bench, and then the second. The spine should remain still with the abdominal muscles bracing during the entire exercise. Repeat this movement, for _____ minute(s). Be sure to breathe normally throughout this exercise.

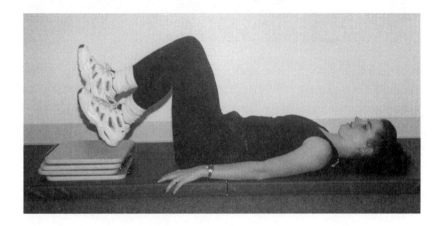

FORM NOTE: If this exercise causes back pain, try bending the knees up further toward the chest and using a higher support for the feet. If it still causes pain, consult the therapist.

2. *Reverse pretzel curls.* With one foot propped on a low bench or other support, cross the other foot over the knee of the propped leg (as shown). Tighten the abdominal muscles and lift both knees toward the chest as you breathe out. Lower the legs slowly

back to the bench and repeat_____ times. Then repeat with
the other leg crossed.

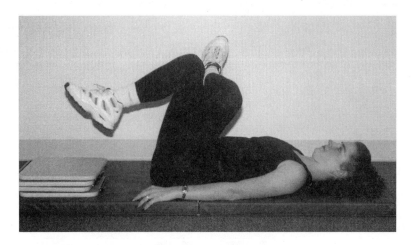

3. *Reverse curl.* Lying on your back, with feet on the floor, tighten
   the abdominal muscles and brace the spine in a neutral position. Then lift both feet up, pulling both knees up toward the
   chest, and slowly lower them back to starting position. Breathe
   out as the feet come up and in as you lower them to the floor.

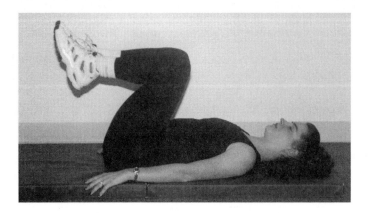

Again, this exercise should not hurt the back. An easier starting position is with the feet propped as in the first two exercises.

Figure 38. Examples of Self-Mobilization Techniques for the Upper and Lower Back.

1. *Upper back stretch using a chair back.* Hands may be behind the head or crossed in front of the chest to opposite shoulder. Breathe in and lean back over the chair, being careful to keep the head directly over the shoulders and not tipped back. Slowly breathe out and try to press the shoulders gently back over the back of the chair. Then return to starting position.

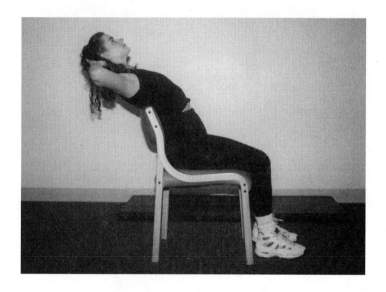

FORM NOTE: If the chair back is not padded, use a towel or pillow for support.

2. *Overall spine stretch.* Start in a seated position with both hands on the thighs. Slowly bend forward sliding the hands down the legs until you reach the feet. Let the head and arms hang down and allow the spine to stretch. Then slowly roll back up, sliding or walking the hands up the legs. The head should come up to starting position last.

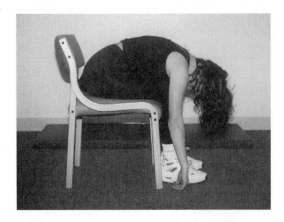

3. *Overall spine stretch, lower back emphasis.* Starting on all fours, slowly sit back with the buttocks moving toward the heels, but not moving the hands. The stretch should be felt in the shoulders as well as the low back.

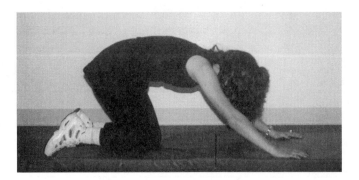

SAMPLE EXERCISE INSTRUCTION SHEETS

These exercise sheets are some that we use frequently with our spine patients. However, many times, we select only some of the exercises on each of several instruction sheets. Examples of these choices are shown in the tables in Figures 27, 28, and 29. Again choices are made based on evaluation findings, with consideration for the specific surgery or procedure. The exercises are recorded on every visit, and a similar sheet can be made for the patient to take home. The patient can usually record their daily exercise on simple graph paper with the exercises written in. This is a helpful reinforcing habit for the first several weeks on an exercise program. It can make a significant impact on the patient if they are given a small exercise log for the year with the clinic name on it.

A sample exercise flow sheet for daily recording of exercise is shown in Figure 39. This form includes some exercises shown in this book and some other exercises we use in our clinic. It is intended as a model only, and individual clinics will need to modify the chart to include all of their exercise options. We use a separate sheet for strength-training exercise done on weight machines.

Figures 40 through 47 are illustrations of some of the exercise instructions we give to our spine patients. The instructions with the illustrations are intended to be given to individuals after they have received more complete instruction in performing the movements. Therefore, the explanations are less detailed than in the exercise illustrations shown in the previous figures.

Figure 40 illustrates Low Back Routine 1. This is a program we use frequently with new patients who need work on back extensor and abdominal recruitment with minimal spinal motion. If patients have position sensitivity to flexion, we will often start with just the first five exercises of this program. If patients are sensitive to extension, we will use numbers 5 through 8. This program is more of

EXERCISE FLOW SHEET

NAME_____

EXERCISE PRECAUTIONS_____ Med Record # _____

DATE																	
INITIALS																	
Treadmill Speed																	
Time																	
Airdyne/Nustep Time																	
Ham Str Sit / Stand																	
Psoas, Pretzel, Piriformis																	
Low Back 1, 2, 3, #_____																	
Cervical Supp / Reg / Isom																	
Wall Ex Mat / Wall																	
UE Aerobics Reg / Back																	
Basic Stab																	
Bridging, Bird Dog																	
Balance, Berg																	
DBugs Reg/Supp, H/K Push																	
Hip Rot Prone / Strap / RBand																	
Funct Act Sit / Lie																	
SLR Lie / Stand / SAQ's / Qsets																	
Squat, Lunge Reg / Stat / Wall																	
Anterior Tib																	
Lying Abs / Oblique																	
RBands UE / LE / Scap / < 90																	
Ribcage #_____																	
Green Sheet Ex 7,8																	
Segm Rotn, Supp LowBack																	
Wand Ex, Pillow Sq UE / LE																	
Gun Str, Single UE Str																	
Ed NS / BS / Booklets																	
Strength																	
Total Gym UE / LE																	
MODALITIES	1	2	3	4	5	6	7	8	9	10	11	12	13	14	15	16	17	18
NOTE :_____																	
1. US 1 / 3 mhz																	
2. ESTIM BP / IFES																	
3. Traction ICT / IPT																	
4. Heat / Ice Therapy																	

Supine   Prone   Side lying   Sitting   Standing

Deep Sweep   Upper/Lower   Cervical   Interscap   Low Back   Hip   Wrist/Hand   Incision

UE   LE   Rotator Cuff   Sacral/Buttock   Knee-Chest   Free Weights   Elng Stretch

Figure 39. Sample Exercise Flow Sheet

a "mid-range" back exercise program and is usually effective for beginning exercise in many patient regimens.

Figure 40. Low Back Routine 1

Do only exercises marked by therapist. Do exercises slowly and breathe normally.

1. Lie on stomach. Tighten buttocks _____ times

2. Lift one arm straight to the back with palm facing the ceiling. Repeat _____ times, alternating arms.

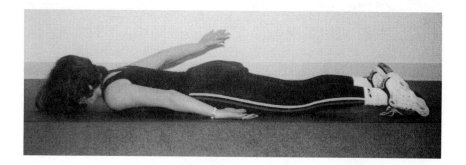

3. Lift one leg no more than a few inches off the mat, then lower slowly. Alternate legs _____ times.

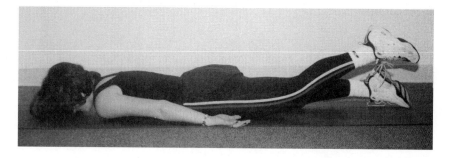

4. Push up into arch position. Try to keep hips on the mat. Hold five seconds and breathe normally. Repeat ____ times.

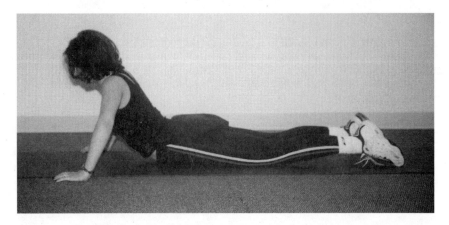

5. Bend knee up toward chest, supporting the thigh with clasped hands. Slowly straighten knee as much as possible. Hold for ten seconds. Repeat and hold fifteen seconds, then repeat and hold thirty seconds. Repeat series on the other leg.

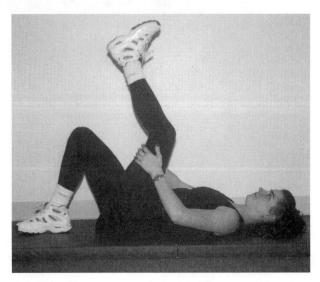

6. On your back with knees bent, tighten abdominals and lift chin toward the ceiling. Repeat _____ times.

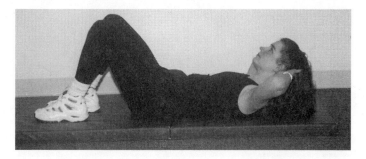

7. Lift buttocks up slowly _____ times.

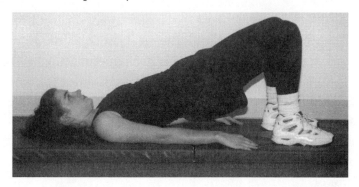

8. On back with knees bent and elbows against the sides and bent at right angles . . .

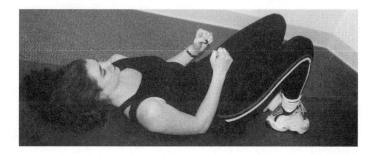

push fists apart and down toward floor _____ times.

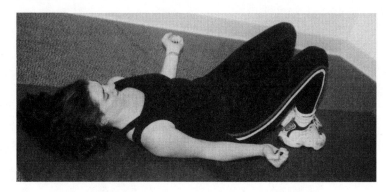

Figure 41 illustrates the patient instruction sheet for our Low Back Routine 2 program. This routine involves more trunk movement and is usually not for a position sensitive patient. Some of the exercises involve a little more intensity, so it is also not recommended as a beginning routine for an individual not familiar with exercise. Because the movements involve most of the range of trunk flexion and extension, we believe that it gives a more active person a chance to recondition core muscles at a variety of lengths and provide some extra support for the spine in that way.

Figure 41. Low Back Routine 2.

Do only exercises marked by therapist. Do exercises slowly and breathe normally.

1. Lift one arm straight to the back with palm facing the ceiling. Repeat _____times, alternating arms.

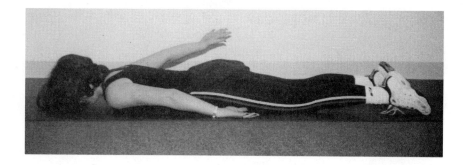

2. Lift one leg no more than a few inches off the mat, then lower slowly. Alternate legs _____ times.

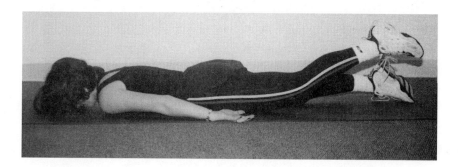

3. With hands at sides on the floor, pull hands toward your feet as you lift head and shoulders slowly _____times.

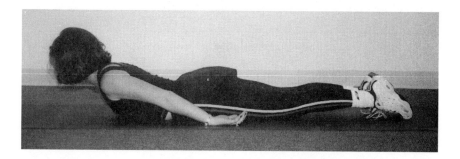

4. With weight supported on forearms and knees as shown, press down on forearms and lift your hips a few inches off the floor. Tighten abdominals so that the back does not arch at all. Repeat ____ times.

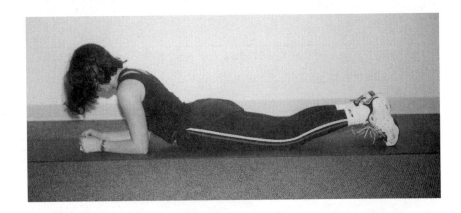

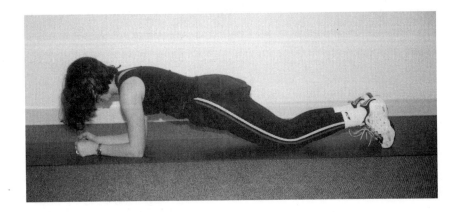

5. Push up into arch position. Try to keep hips on the mat. Hold five seconds and breathe normally. Repeat ____ times.

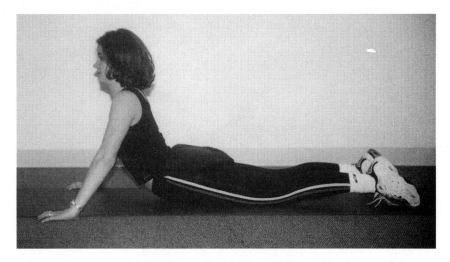

6. Lying on back with knees bent, tighten abdominals and lift chin toward the ceiling. Repeat ____ times.

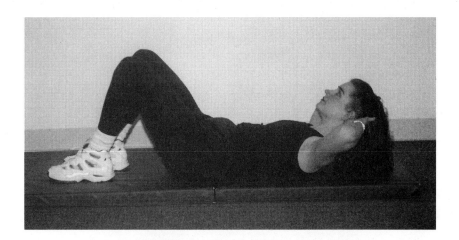

7. With the same position as in #6, lift one knee toward chest while lifting head. Try to touch forehead with knee. Alternate knees ____times.

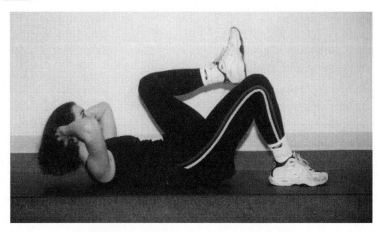

8. Bend knee up toward chest, supporting the thigh with clasped hands. Slowly straighten knee as much as possible. Hold for ten seconds. Repeat and hold fifteen seconds, then repeat and hold thirty seconds. Repeat the series on the other leg.

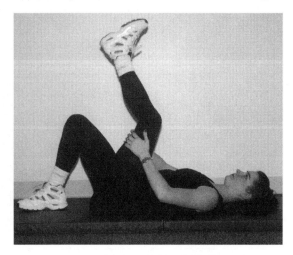

Figure 42 illustrates Low Back Routine 3. This program was designed to exercise trunk muscles with the physioball at a beginner level of difficulty relative to many of the physioball programs that are available now. It is called Low Back 3 because it does require more trunk muscle strength. This program is a good progression step from either Low Back 1 or 2. These exercises are just a few examples of Level II spine stabilization.

We will use this program for younger or more active patients to help them restore their balance and coordination.

Figure 42. Low Back Routine 3.

The first three exercises are done with head and shoulders supported on the ball or foot stool, with the back held in a neutral position throughout. Back, hips, and abdominals should be held tight to maintain a straight spine throughout the exercises.

1. Lift one arm at a time reaching overhead, keeping back from arching. Repeat _____ times, each arm.

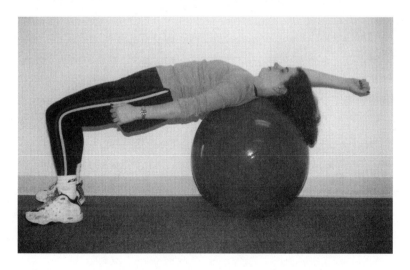

2. Hold arms out to sides at shoulder level. Turn thumbs up as far as possible then down as far as possible _____ times.

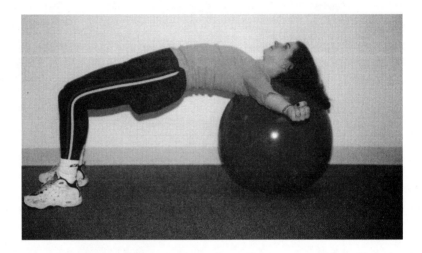

3. With your elbow at sides and arms bent at a right angle, pull the backs of hands toward the floor keeping elbows pressed against sides. Repeat _____ times.

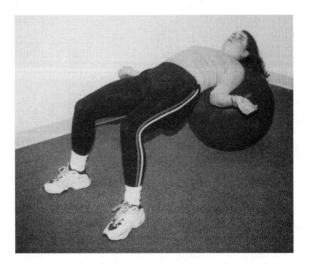

Exercises 4 through 6 are done with support only under the thighs and hands. Pay careful attention to your back position and do not let your back arch or sag. Hold your abdominals tight throughout the exercises.

4. Bend one knee slowly, alternating legs ____ times on each leg.

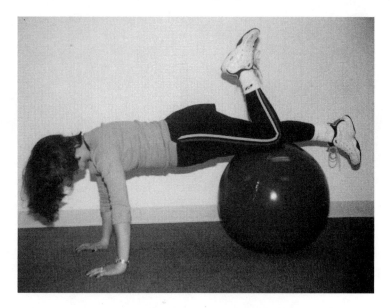

5. Pump ankles, alternating them ____ times each.

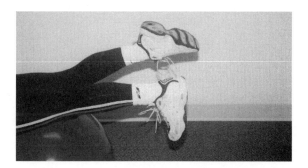

6. Start with legs slightly apart. Press one thigh down and slightly lift the other leg. Alternate legs ____times.

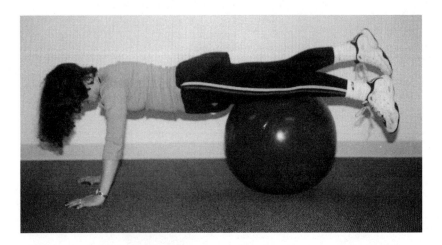

The supported low back exercise patient instruction sheet is shown in Figure 43. These exercises are very good early movements for almost all patients post surgery or procedure. The first exercise is good for pain control and is also a recommended movement to do in the morning to avoid excessive stiffness when first getting out of bed.

The other two exercises are designed to begin to actively work hip rotators in both directions gently.

Figure 43. Supported Low Back Exercises

1. Lie on back with knees bent and feet together. Using small motions, rock knees side to side about two inches only in each direction. You should rock both to right and left once each second. This exercise should not be painful and should be comfortable to do for about two minutes at a time.

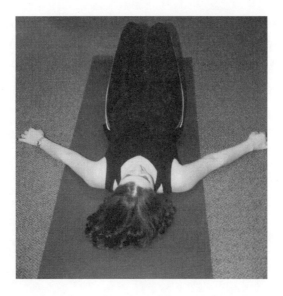

2. Lie on back with knees bent and feet apart. Bend one knee inward toward the other leg as shown, stretching the outer hip of that leg mildly. Repeat this with the other leg _____times per leg.

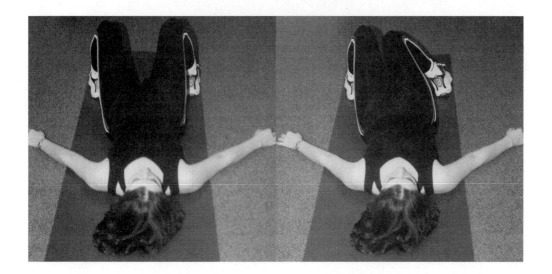

3. Lying on back with knees bent and feet together, slowly move right knee to the side and down toward the floor. Only move each knee out as far as is comfortable. Return to starting position and repeat with the other leg ____times each leg.

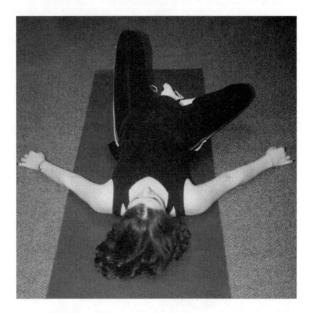

Figure 44. Seated Trunk Circles Stabilization Exercise

This exercise requires no equipment and can be done just about anywhere as a quick muscle tune-up which can be during the day, not necessarily with your regular exercise routine. These movements will fire all of the trunk muscles and wake them up if they have been slacking off during your day!

Sit on a high surface (table, high bed, or kitchen counter) with thighs fully supported, so that when you bend your knees past a right angle, the back of your calves touch the table.

Sit with your back straight, and throughout the exercise pretend your back, shoulders, and head are all glued to a board so that movement will occur only at your hips.

Now imagine that you can write with the top of your head. Draw the largest circles you can with the top of your head with out "coming unglued" from the board or losing your balance. Draw ten circles in one direction, then ten in the other direction. Repeat sets of ten working up to five sets in each direction.

Be sure your posture is perfect throughout the exercise! You may want to watch yourself in the mirror to be sure body parts do not move away from best posture.

Figure 45 shows an example patient education sheet for controlling radiating leg pain. This technique is part of a McKenzie approach (1991). The therapist must first assess whether the method described is effective for the individual. Then, instructions should be fully explained by the therapist first and the sheet can be used as a reference for the patient to take home. The instructions usually need to be reinforced frequently.

Figure 45. Instructions for Controlling Leg Pain.

With onset or flare up of leg pain, it is helpful to repeat this procedure several times per day. If you are unable to decrease the leg pain with these measures, be sure to contact your physical therapist or physician as soon as possible.

Lie face down using pillows under your abdomen if you are unable to lie flat. Remain face down for a few minutes and try to determine if this position helps decrease the leg pain. It may take a few minutes to notice a difference, so it is important not to rush.

If lying face down does not bring relief, try shifting your legs to one side still remaining flat on your stomach. Stay a few minutes if possible, to be sure pressure will not be changed in this position. If no relief occurs, try moving the legs to the other side. Some individuals find that ice on the low back facilitates this process.

If you find a position that decreases the pain, then take the legs back to the center but separate them slightly. Try a slow press up about half way, being sure no leg pain occurs (return to flat lying if leg pain occurs). If the press-up is not painful hold for ten to twenty seconds, then repeat five to ten times.

If this procedure helps decrease the leg pain, then bend backward frequently during the day, emphasizing the movement in the low back. Backward bending may be done standing, sitting with the hands pressing the low back forward, or with the prone press-up. Discuss options with your therapist.

Figures 46 and 47 illustrate some examples of upper body work to integrate into lumbar rehabilitation. This is valuable as it can help facilitate postural muscle recruitment and better overall functional mobility of the spine. These are simple beginner level exercises and should be done where applicable in pain-free ranges of both the neck and shoulders.

Note that extension or backward bending of the neck should be marked as an exercise that should only be done if recommended by the therapist. We usually have older patients, patients with excessive kyphosis, or patients with history of cervical pathology avoid backward bending of the neck. These same patients can benefit from the specific strengthening offered by the example elastic resistance exercises which mostly target the posterior shoulder girdle, as well as the upper extremities, to help posture as well as to augment spine stabilization.

At times, patients may have enough painful movement with the lower body or may be at a stage where they need to restrict the movement of the lower body. Upper body exercise is particularly helpful in these cases. Of course upper body strength is an integral part of physical conditioning in any case, but at times it can fit in as a strategy to allow a patient to exercise successfully in one area when he or she is having difficulty activating other areas.

Figure 46. Cervical Motion Exercises

All exercises should be done with good posture and very little movement in the shoulders, upper or lower back. Starting position for each exercise is a *neutral neck* position with the head directly over the shoulders, level chin, and looking straight ahead. These exercises should all be done slowly and should not be painful!

1. *Flexion.* Bend head forward pressing chin toward chest. Return to starting neutral position and repeat _____times.

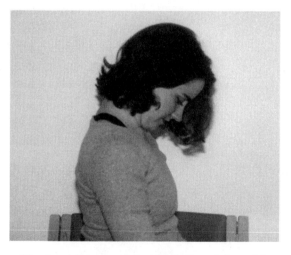

2. *Extension. Check with your therapist before doing this exercise. This movement should be avoided by some individuals.* With neck supported with your hand, slowly tip your head back and look up at the ceiling. Return to neutral position and repeat _____ times.

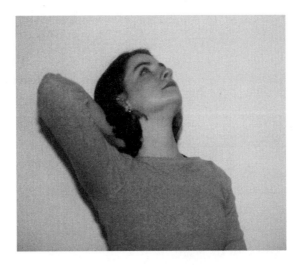

3. *Lateral.* Bend head to the side bringing the ear toward the shoulder. Be sure not to let the head tip back at all. Return to neutral position. Repeat to the other side for ____ times to each side.

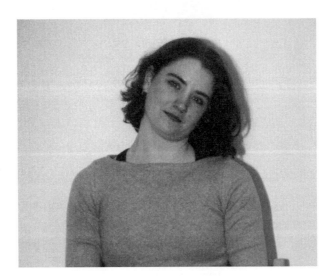

4. Rotation. Turn head slowly as far as possible to one side. Be sure the chin does not lift at all. Repeat to the other side for ____ times for each side.

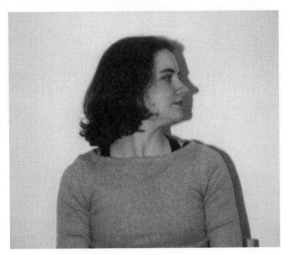

5. Three way shrugs. Start standing or seated with arms straight down at sides. 1) Lift shoulders up towards ears.

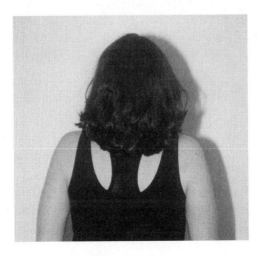

5. 2) Pull shoulder blades back and down.

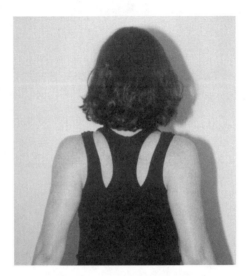

5. 3) Lower both shoulders down and stretch arms down toward the floor. Repeat this sequence _____ times.

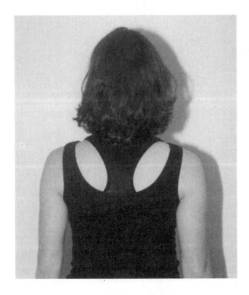

Figure 47. Upper Body Strengthening
with Elastic Resistance

When using elastic resistance try to hold the band at a length that gives you challenging resistance throughout the movement. But do not hold the band with too much tension. You should be able to do smooth continuous movements without jerking.

1. *Lat (latissimus) pulldown.* Start with the band overhead with hands about shoulder-width distance apart. With elbows bent slightly, pull arms down and out to sides as shown. Slowly return to starting position. Repeat _____ times.

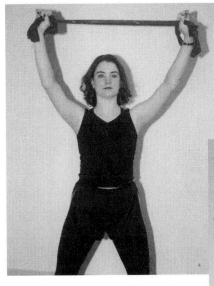

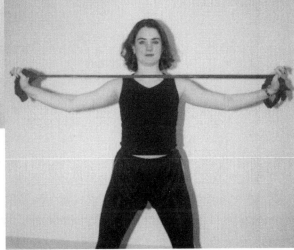

2. *Bow and arrow.* Hold band in left hand with arm straight out to the side. Grasp band with the right hand about twelve inches away, as shown. Pull right hand back to the right shoulder, keeping the left arm straight. Repeat _____ times, then repeat series on the other side.

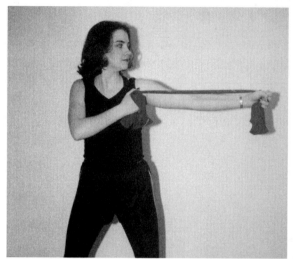

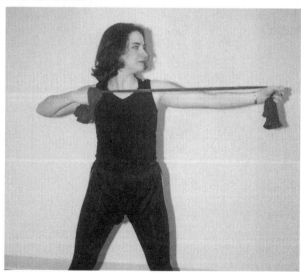

3. *Side to side.* Hold the band in front of you at shoulder level with hands shoulder width distance apart. Straighten one arm out to the side then return to starting position. Repeat with the other arm, alternating arms doing each _____ times. You can also do this exercise lying down.

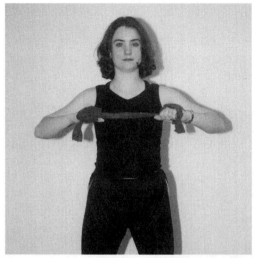

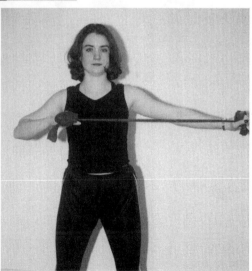

4. *Diagonal behind the back.* Grasp band as shown, with thumb of top hand pointing down and thumb of lower hand pointing up. Extend top arm up and lower arm down, then slowly return to starting position. Repeat _____ times, then change arms and repeat series.

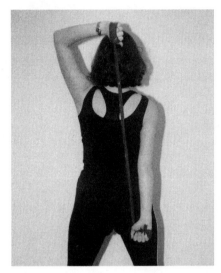

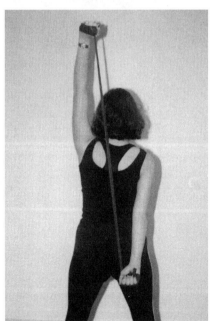

Chapter 11

•,,••❶•,,,,,•••••

Protocol Development

Currently, physical therapy is a combination of art, science, and gambling. Although there is more science available to utilize in our interventions, the method of delivery often determines the amount of success. Method of delivery is the art form, and refers to the therapist's capability to relate to individual patients so they take responsibility for making the needed changes. Science is used to accurately identify the needed changes in the rehabilitation process, and unfortunately this still involves a lot of gambling.

The physical therapy profession has been making strides toward improving the scientific component of our practice and this can be seen most recently in the *Guide to Physical Therapist Practice, Second Edition* (American Physical Therapy Association [APTA] 2001). The *Guide* is designed as a comprehensive, extensively peer-reviewed resource for all of the assessment and treatment options available in each diagnostic category. The *Guide* ensures that all possibilities can be considered in a given treatment scenario, and its list of choices is intended to be exhaustive. Our protocols, in contrast, are designed to focus on some specific selections within the recommended choices. All of our protocol choices can be found within the *Guide,* and have been chosen with attention to addressing conditions often found following a given lumbar spine procedure.

We believe that considering the effects of the procedure on each type of tissue involved is one way all structures can be rehabilitated maximally. In the next sections, we give some examples of tissue areas and how the *Guide* provides additional details for treatment of that area. Clinicians often find it difficult to revise their treatments when a patient fails to respond as expected. By trying to troubleshoot by suspected problem tissue, the *Guide* can provide alternate management ideas for that area.

FURTHER DEVELOPMENT OF LUMBAR SPINE PROTOCOLS

The focus of this book has been on developing rehabilitation to augment various procedures performed on the lumbar spine. We have combined treatments designed to address the many problems of patients following lumbar spine procedures. Practitioners working with our protocols may find variations in their patients' responses. Working with the *Guide* along with our protocols might help practitioners further modify our protocols to take into account their own situations and the responses of their patients.

The *Guide* gives detailed preferred practice patterns in four major categories: musculoskeletal, neuromuscular, cardiovascular/pulmonary, and integumentary. We have tried to emphasize throughout the book that all four of these categories are important to consider when caring for a patient following spine surgery. This may be the first deterrent to a therapist who is interested in working with these patients. It is just too complicated! But when we realize that no one has all of the answers regarding patient care (of this or any other patient group), we can be glad that a large armamentarium is available for designing programs which will improve the patient's condition. The *Guide* can serve as a source for alternative treatment choices, especially if the clinician is able to pinpoint an individual patient's problem within one of the four areas.

POSTSURGICAL CARE ON A TISSUE BY TISSUE BASIS

Following surgery on the lumbar spine, there are several tissues of interest in the therapy program (McFarland 1994). This has been addressed in several places in the book, but will be recapped here, also providing some suggestions for utilizing the *Guide* as well as giving ideas needing investigation. Only a few tissues will be discussed as examples, and ways to apply the *Guide* should become evident simply with its use.

DISC PROTECTION

There is a specific preferred practice pattern, Pattern I of the Musculoskeletal section, for "Impaired Joint Mobility, Motor Function, Muscle Performance, and Range of Motion Associated with Bony or Soft Tissue Surgery" (APTA 2001, 277-86) . The diagnostic categories listed refer to the pathologies for which the surgeries are done, but the *Guide* does not differentiate much between surgeries. There are several recommendations for manual therapy, exercise, and ergonomics which can all function to protect the disc. The lists given in these patterns are exhaustive and the therapist is responsible for narrowing down the choices. Choices would vary considerably depending on the surgical intervention. A subject for future research and a suggestion for the next edition of the *Guide* is to determine which choices tend to fit with which surgeries.

It seems logical, but has yet to be addressed in the literature, that the same precautions used trying to resolve a disc problem nonsurgically, apply initially after a disc surgery, so the disc can heal without reherniation. Reinforced posture and support for the spine are important, and recruitment of stabilizing musculature for the lumbar segments would be priorities for protection of the newly operated disc. In our protocols, we identify means of providing disc protection. If these fail for a given patient, the therapist can turn to Preferred Practice Pattern I in the *Guide* for alternative choices.

LIGAMENTOUS STATUS AND JOINT MOBILITY

Ideas might be obtained from the same Pattern I for addressing the recovery of ligamentous function in the lumbar spine. However, more options may be found for this aspect of care under Pattern F of the Musculoskeletal section, which is entitled "Impaired Joint Mobility, Motor Function, Muscle Performance, Range of Motion, and Reflex Integrity Associated with Spinal Disorders" (APTA 2001, 223-9). Working to address both the shortened or scarred ligaments, as well as those which are weakened and potentially unstable, is important for the majority of postsurgical spine patients. However, the unknown factor is how recovery of ligamentous function, which eventually will involve movement, can safely integrate with the priority we have established for protecting the intervertebral discs. Remember that protecting the disc may involve avoiding movement for a period of time. The ligaments may have to be addressed in different time frames postsurgically, depending on the surgery. We acknowledge that specific ligament problems may not be identifiable in the lumbar spine, but that restricted or excessive level-by-level mobility in the vertebrae indicates need for attention. Mobility of the lumbar spine may be a factor to consider after a few weeks of recovery in nonfusion surgeries. Stability, and not mobility, must usually remain the focus for several weeks following fusions.

Because the discs also have some tissue and characteristics of ligaments, we need to look at both areas together in many situations. Some important research questions for the future include:

1. How much movement is needed to optimize ligamentous function in each area of the spine? Do we need to analyze the need for movement of each intervertebral level separately because of the differences in each level's configuration?

2. Can movement of the ligaments affect disc health? Are there forces and movements which can actually improve the health of both tissues, and if so, what are these forces?

3. Can the ligaments adjacent to the fused spine levels be *strengthened*, better protecting the function and disc integrity at these levels?

4. What is the optimal amount of movement and force to produce the best longevity of the ligaments and discs of the spine?

BONE INTEGRITY

Although bone integrity is primarily an area of concern with patients following fusion surgery, it may also be a factor with any elderly patient undergoing spinal procedures. Preferred Practice Pattern A of the Musculoskeletal section, "Primary Prevention/Risk Reduction for Skeletal Demineralization" can be the resource for protocol components in this area (APTA 2001, 141-51). This can be a forgotten area in patient care following other spine procedures, and once again the therapist is in the ideal position to insure that bone integrity is addressed. As we have pointed out in other areas of the book, bone integrity is a consideration for many of the patients if they have nutritional problems, if they smoke, if they take certain medications which impair calcium absorption, or if they have a very slender build. Considerations of these factors in the rehabilitation, as well as consulting with the physician regarding nutritional and medication management, can help overcome bone problems. Left unaddressed, lack of bone integrity can be a factor in "failed back syndrome".

MUSCLE PERFORMANCE

This is an area of emphasis in our protocols. There are suggestions throughout all four sections of the *Guide* which should help with choices for identified muscle performance problems. Some patients may be helped most with a practice pattern for muscle perform-ance from the Neuromuscular section, especially when changes have occurred in the neurological status. The neuromuscular ap-proach is also often helpful to a patient who is unfamiliar with ex-ercise and may need more attention in order to follow movement instructions. Some patients may benefit from exercise choices in a preferred practice pattern from the Cardiovascular section first, if the patient's primary limitation is endurance. All of the sections suggest active rehabilitation for the muscular component of prob-lems throughout the body. We have tried narrowing the scope of choices for working on muscle performance in this book, in order to demonstrate our thought processes in dealing with specific pa-tient scenarios. We have stressed the importance of critical atten-tion to all exercise selection. Again, if our thought process does not work for particular therapists or their patients, the *Guide* is a good place to turn for ideas.

SUMMARY

In this book, we describe practice for several specific conditions and procedures used in lumbar spine disorders. At this point, working with rehabilitation of the spine, we limit the choices in our treat-ment descriptions, providing the possibility for a reproducible pro-gram. We hope by doing this, other clinicians will try these specific programs and will be able to help research the efficacy of the program components. As we have mentioned before, these protocols are a starting point for a more refined system in the future.

We will need to look at outcomes for the patients and modify the rehabilitation so outcomes for patients improve with time. Jette & Jette (1997) point out in some of their outcome work that therapists have the most uncertainty in their treatment choices when working with spine pathologies. We understand this uncertainty, as so much of the spine literature is still controversial and basically inconclusive. These factors make therapists' attempts to describe specific practice intimidating and also, very likely subject to considerable criticism. However, our intent has been to describe our rationale for treatment choices so others may use the ideas, eventually leading to a body of practices that have been tested with results documented.

When therapeutic choices that appear to make positive changes in a majority of patients following surgery become apparent, they can be reported to academic institutions or to those who are equipped to do controlled studies. The clinicians are needed for this critical first step. We can report our outcomes to the institutions along with our description of a certain program component. The controlled studies of a given component can follow. And we will be another step closer to a more successful care path for our patients. It is helpful and encouraging to realize that the rehabilitation profession is most likely best positioned to monitor the most aspects of recovery from spine surgery.

Physical therapy treatments for spine patients still have a relatively high failure rate, although no studies can actually give us a solid statistic on that.

With a willingness to share treatment experiences and ideas, we can apply lessons learned to the next set of protocols. We limited our emphasis in this text to the lumbar spine, to keep the work manageable. Now that this first step is complete, we plan to go on

to the cervical and thoracic spine procedures and continue working on refining the lumbar protocols as described. We are interested in having more co-workers in this effort. We would love to
have input from as many clinicians as possible and would welcome
your comments and ideas:

Carol McFarland, Don Burkhart
P.O. Box 7157
Tyler, TX75711
mcf1@gower.net

Appendix

●●●●●●●●●●●●●

Rehabilitation of Patients Undergoing Spine Surgery in the Eyes of Physicians, Patients, and Payers: A Physical Therapy Challenge.

—Carol M. McFarland MS PT OCS, 1998

Care and management of the patient with spine disorders is a subject fraught with controversy in both the surgical and nonsurgical arenas (Atlas et al.1996; Cherkin et al. 1996; Deyo and Phillips 1996; Ibarra 1997; Keller et al. 1996). Spine surgeries are done twice as often in the United States, compared to most developed countries, yet the care and follow-up of the patients undergoing surgery is widely variable with variable outcomes and little agreement on methods (Atlas et al.1996; Deyo and Phillips 1996; Malter et al. 1998; Nykvist et al. 1995; Taylor et al. 1996). Many surgical articles refer to rehabilitation following spine surgery, but surgeons are not in agreement about its use (Carragee, Helms, and O'Sullivan 1996; Mayer et al. 1998). Some surgical reports focusing on outcome do not discuss the path to the outcome, especially regarding follow-up care. The author's experience in evaluating and providing physical

therapy for over two thousand postoperative spine patients identi-
fies problems with inconsistent use of rehabilitation between surgeons and within individual surgeon's caseloads. Additionally, there
is some hesitancy for patients to participate in rehabilitation if they
have previously been to a physician who has any doubts about exercise or activity. The literature shows a relative lack of empirical
evidence for the more commonly acceptable rehabilitation methods for nonsurgical spine problems (Cherkin et al. 1996; Faas 1996;
Jette and Jette 1997). This, in addition to spine surgeons' lack of
agreement on the use of postoperative therapy, presents a problem
with acceptance of rehabilitation in the eyes of some physicians and
patients and in turn creates a challenge in obtaining reimburse-
ment. The purpose of this paper is to review the literature on postoperative care for the spine patient with regard to outcomes and
the challenge of justification of rehabilitation for physicians, patients, and payers. There were no papers found which addressed
this challenge specifically, so three categories of papers were chosen for review of the following aspects of the above purpose: out-
comes-research on spine surgeries which may directly or indirectly
support or refute rehabilitation, studies with reference to particular payers, and studies describing and/or comparing types of rehabilitation parameters to help better identify which therapies are
most effective.

OUTCOME STUDIES SUPPORTING REHABILITATION FOR THE POSTSURGICAL SPINE PATIENTS

Hinkley and Jaremko (1997) carried out an unusual study showing
positive postoperative outcomes of ninety-one percent on workers'
compensation patients, and gave a fairly detailed description of the
postoperative rehabilitation following "360" lumbar fusion starting the
day after surgery. Often workers' compensation patients are described

as having the poorest prognosis with lumbar problems (Cherkin et al. 1996; Elam et al. 1997; Mayer et al. 1998; Taylor et al. 1996). There have been a few studies by rehabilitation specialists also describing workers' compensation patients showing favorable outcome with aggressive "functional restoration" treatment done with tertiary level patients, but they do not address the early care or specific adaptations needed for specific surgical problems (Curtis, Mayer, and Gatchel 1994; Mayer et al. 1998). Curtis, Mayer & Gatchel showed that postdiscectomy patients, both male and female, showed greater isokinetic lifting forces than nonoperative lumbar patients, possibly adding to the argument that strength is an important issue to address with spine patients.

There have been a few, but not many, studies emphasizing the importance of rehabilitation in postoperative spine care. Manniche et al. (1993) described dynamic back exercises which were used after lumbar discectomy with success. Brennan et al. (1994) showed that oxygen consumption was more than three times as important as any other single variable in differentiating between good and poor outcome following lumbar microdiscectomy. These studies, provide evidence for specific postoperative rehabilitation from a movement control perspective, a strength perspective, and an aerobic perspective. It is somewhat of a conflict that most orthopedic surgeries for extremities strongly emphasize the need for rehabilitation, but that rehabilitation is an area of *de*-emphasis in spine surgeries. The spine surgeries would seemingly require *more* rehabilitation for recovery from not only the musculoskeletal component of the surgery, but from the neurologic component as well (Manniche et al. 1993; Silhoven et al. 1997; Potvin and O'Brien 1998). In fact, due to the increased involvement of the neurologic symptoms with some spine surgeries, many patients report immediate, dramatic relief once an offending nerve is decompressed. This encourages both the grateful patient and the surgeon to want to leave "well-enough alone" and not think about restoration of the musculoskeletal component that could have helped ensure maximal capability to return to activity safely (McFarland 1994).

STUDIES SHOWING SUBOPTIMAL OUTCOMES WITH SPINE SURGERY POPULATIONS

Studies showing suboptimal surgical results for spine patients point to a need for evaluation of clinical paths used (Ibarra 1997). Rehabilitation may be a very important area for improving the clinical path, both preoperatively and postoperatively. A large study of 6376 patients in Washington State described surgeries done in 1988 with a five year follow-up (Malter et al. 1998). They showed reoperation rate was the same for fusion and for nonfusion patients, but the complication rate was eighteen percent for fusion patients and seven percent for nonfusion patients. Examination of the clinical paths might identify areas where these patients could have had improvements in follow-up. In studies of this magnitude, rehabilitation is often not addressed, and the question remains if rehabilitation done on a consistent basis may have changed these rates. A Finnish study in 1995 showed a thirteen year follow-up on patients who were hospitalized for severe sciatica (Nykvist et al. 1998). Two hundred and twenty of these patients were treated surgically and 122 were treated conservatively with outcomes at one, five, and thirteen years. At thirteen years, sixteen percent of the surgical group had undergone reoperation, fourteen percent of the conservative group had surgery, and nearly seventy percent of the entire population still had sciatica, and forty percent had retired on disability pensions. Cherkin et al. (1996) contend that some of the problem lies in the impression that the initial onset of back pain is something that will resolve completely in most patients and thus it is not worked up appropriately in primary care. In Cherkin's study of 219 patients making an initial visit for lumbar pain to a primary physician, he found only sixty-seven percent reported good outcomes after seven weeks, and seventy-one percent were satisfied with their condition a year later. The American Academy of Orthopaedic Surgeons (1990) asserted the now often-quoted statement that "ninety percent of patients with back pain seen in general practice will be pain free within three months" (no matter what you do or don't do for them). Some clinicians feel strongly that we need to re-evaluate our management of these initial patients, pay more attention to their potential long term problems, and create more detailed clinical paths.

Deyo and Phillips (1996) describe the dilemma of the wide and varied research in spine care, with three challenges which more than likely are key for all clinicians dealing with these patients: 1) better diagnostic strategies and classifications for the spine patients; 2) better theory explaining episodes of nonspecific low back pain; and 3) more methodological rigor for testing nonsurgical treatments. They point out that the conflicting and competing theories frustrate the practitioners and the patients, as well as diminish our credibility as spine specialists. Therapists echo these concerns in many of their studies in trying to describe care for specific dysfunctions in spine patients (DeLitto et al. 1993; Fitzgerald et al. 1994; Jette and Jette 1997; McFarland 1994; Rothhaupt et al. 1997).

OUTCOME STUDIES REFUTING THE USE OF REHABILITATION FOR POSTOPERATIVE SPINE PATIENTS

The cover page of the widely read *BACK Letter* (1996) asked the question recently "Will Exercise Survive as a Treatment for Low Back Pain in the Cost-Conscious World of Managed Care?" The article was referring to a Dutch study refuting exercise for *acute* low back pain (Faas 1996). The study actually supported use of exercise for subacute and chronic pain, but the *BACK Letter* article went on to describe exercise as an expense which could be saved by sending the patient to a health club. The Faas study critiqued some previous exercise studies and concluded that many of them were insufficient in providing evidence supporting the use of exercise at all for the acute spine patient.

Carragee, Helms, and O'Sullivan (1996) have started a line of research in which patients are given no postoperative restrictions following lumbar discectomy and are urged to go back to work and regular activity as soon as possible following the surgery. In the published study of this project, fifty patients showed good outcomes with pain relief and work capability out to two year follow-up. Carragee made a presentation at the American Back Society meeting (1997) of further work with 120 patients in this regimen. He explained that postoperative treatment tended to "medicalize" the surgery, giving the patient the impression that they were more disabled than they actually were and, for that reason, risks outweighed the benefits of a formal postoperative physical therapy program.

The above studies were carefully done and have made valid points against rehabilitation. However, some of the conclusions may be based on an incomplete perception of what is done in rehabilitation for patients in general, but especially for the population of spine patients. Probably one of the best descriptive guides explaining the scope and thought process of the physical therapy treatments is found in the recent *Guide to Physical Therapist Practice* (American Physical Therapy Association, 1997). These might be utilized in educating referring physicians, patients, or payers to best explain what role therapy can play in recovery from spine surgery. Different types of spine surgeries fit within several of the preferred practice patterns in the "Musculoskeletal Treatment Guides". However, Jette and Jette (1997) point out another problem among therapists treating the spine patients based on outcome work with Focus on Therapeutic Outcomes (FOTO) database. The therapists showed more uncertainty with treatment choices for spine patients than with other orthopedic patients. Jette and Jette concluded that physical therapy practice may be influenced by "idiosyncratic factors" with clinical decision making, which sheds an unfavorable light on therapists as decision makers for spine patients. This study was done before the publication of the *Guide* which may now reduce some of the therapists' uncertainty.

STUDIES WITH REFERENCE TO PAYERS

With Medicare going to the prospective payment system (PPS), opportunities for rehabilitation for the Medicare postoperative spine patients appear to be best in an inpatient setting, since outpatient therapy is generally more restricted. Clinical paths may need to be adjusted for the Medicare patient with more inpatient emphasis and possible use of SNF beds or home health. For many of the older postoperative spine patients, this may represent a more appropriate level of care than the previous, often inadequate treatment which was given on an outpatient basis under the previous Medicare cap of $900. Many times the patient was simply sent home and their function not addressed beyond household ambulation. The Medicare system has been subject to a lot of abuse and reports of large scale problems point to the need for reform within Medicare's payment system in general and specifically for rehabilitation (Chan et al. 1997; Sutton, DeJong, and Wilkerson 1996).

Sutton et al. (1996) proposed a conceptual model for payment similar to Diagnostic Related Groupings (DRG's) which would be more incentive-driven than PPS, which would reward providers with better outcomes. The system would withhold a "fixed proportion" of the DRG-like payment and place it in a "quality of care" pool, which would be distributed to the facilities with a "predesignated facility-level, case-mix-adjusted outcomes."

Workers' compensation has already been mentioned in both positive and negative studies. The fact seems to remain that generally workers' compensation patients are less likely to do well, are more likely to have surgery, and are more likely to have repeat surgery (Elam et al. 1997; Taylor et al. 1996). The articles which report success with the workers' compensation population all emphasize importance of the functional restoration through complete rehabilitation in obtaining good outcomes with these patients (Curtis, Mayer, and Gatchel 1994; Hinkley and Jaremko 1997). It is now up to the therapists to be sure that the communication with the compensation providers and employers includes evidence such as these studies.

With regard to managed care, Fletchall and Hickerson (1997) outlined the therapist's responsibilities in assuring that their patients can fulfill the needed rehabilitation for optimal recovery. These include interaction with patient, MCOs, employers, and case managers; clinical skills which shift responsibility to the patient for full active participation in their recovery; and communication and presentation of our data on outcomes. That is a substantial responsibility and may appear overwhelming to therapists as a whole. However, by concentrating and recording activity with interaction and shifting responsibility, the outcome information may make itself more apparent.

STUDIES DESCRIBING AND COMPARING ASPECTS OF REHABILITATION FOR THE POSTOPERATIVE SPINE

There are many basic science studies examining forces on various tissues of the spine and the possible changes which may occur as a result. Some of these studies can help make a case for applying these forces during therapy to help promote spine stabilization or to protect the spine from mechanical abnormalities (Hides, Richardson, and Jull 1996; Potvin and O'Brien 1998; Silhoven et al. 1997). Other studies give kinematic information of the effects of surgery, especially fusion, which can help us better select movements to target the fusion area completely with regard to muscle recruitment (Yoganandan et al. 1993). It is debatable whether basic science studies should be generalized into the creation of rehabilitation programs, but they can certainly add to the rationale for treatment choices.

There have been some very good outcome studies on the effects of therapy itself in resolving disc symptoms. Functional improvements for the spine patient have been correlated with many different therapies (Curtis, Mayer, and Gatchel 1994; DeLitto et al. 1993; Donelson, Silva and Murphy 1990; Fitzgerald et al. 1994; Manniche et al. 1993; Rothhaupt et al. 1997; Saal and Saal 1989). It is not within the scope of this paper to review all of these studies as there are numerous ones for all conservative venues. However, it is important to have information on components of individual clinical pathways.

SUMMARY

The Maine Lumbar Spine Study with its subjects numbering in the thousands was created in an attempt to clear up confusion and vague terminology surrounding spine disorders and as well as to clarify the point at which a nonsurgical case will do best as a surgical case (Atlas et al. 1996; Keller et al. 1996). The confusion and controversy still exist, as described by Deyo and Phillips (1996), who state "another problem is that much back pain management historically has been a series of fads and fashions." The trend however, is very definitely toward consistency in the treatment decision making and delivery. Physical therapists will continually need to educate physicians, patients, and payers about the therapists' capabilities to accelerate the patient's course down the clinical path, to function in case management for the postoperative patient, being able to monitor progress of all aspects of the patient's recovery: neurologic, integumentary, musculoskeletal, and cardiovascular. The therapist can act as a physician extender, since they see the patient most frequently and can do some of the triage functions for the surgeon. The studies are coming in with increasing numbers of journals: *Spine,* which has gone to bi-weekly publication and has increasing numbers of articles regarding rehabilitation; *Journal of Rehabilitation Outcomes Measures,* a relatively new journal; *Physiotherapy Research International; Medicine and Science in Sports and Exercise,* and of course *Physical Therapy* are just a few of the available resources for therapists. The work still has to be done, but there appears to be better potential than ever to have the physical therapist considered as an integral part of the spine surgery professional team.

References

American Academy of Orthopaedic Surgeons. 1990. *Orthopaedic knowledge update 3: Home study syllabus.* Park Ridge, IL: American Academy of Orthopaedic Surgeons.

American College of Sports Medicine (ACSM). 1991. *Guidelines for exercise testing and prescription, 4th edition.* Philadelphia: Lea & Febiger.

American College of Sports Medicine (ACSM). 1995. *Guidelines for exercise testing and prescription, 5th edition.* Baltimore: Williams and Wilkins.

American Medical Association. 1988. *Guides to evaluation of permanent impairment, 3rd edition.* Chicago: American Medical Association.

American Physical Therapy Association. 1997. Guide to physical therapist practice. *Phys Ther* 77.

American Physical Therapy Association. 2001. Guide to physical therapist practice, Second edition. *Phys Ther* 81.

Atlas, S.J., R.A. Deyo, R.B. Keller, A.M. Chapin, D.L. Patrick, J.M. Long, and D.E. Singer. 1996. The Maine lumbar spine study, part II: 1-year outcomes of surgical and nonsurgical management of sciatica. *Spine* 21: 1777–1786.

———. 1996. The Maine lumbar spine study, part III: 1-year outcomes of surgical and nonsurgical management of lumbar spinal stenosis. *Spine* 21: 1787–94.

Atlas, S.J., R.A. Deyo, D.L. Patrick, K. Convery, R. B. Keller, and D. E. Singer. 1996. The Quebec Task Force classification for spinal disorders and the severity, treatment, and outcomes of sciatica and lumbar spinal stenosis. *Spine* 21: 2885–92.

BACKLetter. 1996. Hagerstown, MD: Lippincott-Raven Publishers.

Basmajian, J., and R. Nyberg. 1993. *Rational manual therapies.* Baltimore: William and Wilkins.

Biondi, Beverly. 1991. Functional stabilization training for low back disorders. Course presented in Tyler, Texas.

Blankenship, K. 1990. *Industrial rehabilitation. A seminar syllabus.* American Therapeutics, Inc.

Borenstein, D., and S. Weisel. 1989. *Low back pain.* Philadelphia: W.B. Saunders Company.

Brennan, G.P., B.B. Schulz, R.S. Hood, J.C. Zahniser, S.C. Johnson, and A.H. Gerber. 1994. The effects of aerobic exercise after lumbar microdiscectomy. *Spine* 19: 735–739.

Carragee, E.J. 1997. Very early return to work of the postoperative discectomy patient, with no specific restrictions; Review of 120 clinical cases from the Stanford University Spine Center. Presentation at American Back Society annual conference: "Diagnosis and Treatment of Neck and Back Pain: The Integrated Approach."

Carragee, E.J., E. Helms, and G.S. O'Sullivan. 1996. Are postoperative activity restrictions necessary after posterior lumbar discectomy? A prospective study of outcomes in 50 consecutive cases. *Spine* 21: 1893–7.

Chan, L., T.D. Koepsell, R.A. Deyo, P.C. Esselman, J.K. Haselkorn, J.K. Lowery, and W.C. Stolov. 1997. The effect of Medicare payment system for rehabilitation hospitals on length of stay, charges, and total payments. *N Engl J Med* 337: 978–85.

Cherkin, D.C., R.A. Deyo, J.H. Street, and L. Barlow. 1996. Predicting poor outcomes for back pain seen in primary care using patients' own criteria. *Spine* 21: 2900–7.

Corrigan, B., and G.D. Maitland. 1985. *Practical Orthopaedic Medicine.* London:Butterworth, 259–263.

Curtis, L., T. Mayer, and R. Gatchel. 1994. Physical progress and residual impairment quantification after functional restoration. *Spine* 19: 401–5.

Cyriax J. 1980. *Textbook of orthopaedic medicine, Volume II: Treatment by manipulation, massage and injection.* London: Bailliere Tindall.

Delitto, A., M.T. Cibulka, R. Erhard, R.W. Bowling, and J.A. Tenhula. 1993. Evidence for use of an extension-mobilization category in acute low back pain syndrome; a prescriptive validation study. *Phys Ther* 73: 216–23.

Deyo, R.A. and W.R. Phillips. 1996. Low back pain. A primary care challenge.
Spine 21: 2826–32.

Donelson, R., G. Silva, and K. Murphy. 1990. Centralization phenomenon: Its usefulness in evaluating and treating referred pain. *Spine* 15: 211–213.

Dreyer, S.J., P.H. Dreyfuss, and A. Cole. 1994. Zygapophysial joint injections. In Weinstein S. (ed.) *Injection techniques: Physical medicine and rehabilitation clinics of North America.* Philadelphia: W.B. Saunders Company.

Dreyfuss, P.H., S.J. Dreyer, and S.A. Herring. 1995. Lumbar zygapophysial (facet) joint injections. *Spine* 21: 2594–2602.

Dreyfuss, P.H., F. Lagattuta, B. Kaplansky, and B. Heller. 1994. Zygapophysial joint injection techniques in the spinal axis. In Lennard TA. (ed.) *State of the art reviews in physical medicine and rehabilitation.* Hanley & Belfus, Inc.

Elam, K., V. Taylor, M.A. Ciol, G.M. Franklin, and R.A. Deyo. 1997. Impact of a worker's compensation practice guideline on lumbar spine fusion in Washington State. *Med Care* 35: 417–24.

Faas, A. 1996. Exercises: Which ones are worth trying, for which patients, and when? *Spine* 21: 2874–9.

Fitzgerald, G.K., P.W. McClure, P. Beattie, and D. Riddle. 1994. Issues in determining treatment effectiveness in manual therapy. *Phys Ther* 74: 227–233.

Fletchall, S., and W.L. Hickerson. 1997. Managed health care: therapist responsibilities. *J Burn Care Rehabil* 18: 61–3.

Gill, K.P., and M.J. Callaghan. 1998. The measurement of lumbar proprioception in individuals with and without low back pain. *Spine* 23: 371–377.

Greenman, P.E. 1996. *Principles of manual medicine. 2nd edition.* Baltimore: Williams & Wilkins.

Hides, J.A., C.A. Richardson, and G.A. Jull. 1996. Multifidus muscle recovery is not automatic after resolution of acute, first episode low back pain. *Spine* 21: 2763–2769.

Hinkley, B.S., and M.E. Jaremko. 1997. Effects of 360-degree fusion in a workers' compensation population. *Spine* 22: 312–323.

Hoeger, W.W.K. 1986. *Lifetime physical fitness and wellness. A personalized program, 2nd edition.* Englewood, Colorado: Morton Publishing Co.

Ibarra, V.L. 1997. Spine update: Clinical pathways. *Spine* 22: 352–357.

Jette, D.U., and A.M. Jette. 1997. Professional uncertainty and treatment choices by physical therapists. *Arch Phys Med Rehabil* 78: 1346–51.

Keller, R.B., S.J. Atlas, D.E. Singer, A.M. Chapin, N.A. Mooney, D.L. Patrick, and R.A. Deyo. 1996. The Maine Lumbar Spine Study, Part I. Background and Concepts. *Spine* 21: 1769–1775.

Kornberg C, and T. McCarthy. 1992. The effects of neural stretching techniques on sympathetic outflow to the lower limbs. *J Orthop Sports Phys Ther* 16.

Lechner, D.E., S.F. Bradbury, and L.A. Bradley. 1998. Detecting sincerity of effort: a summary of methods and approaches. *Phys Ther* 78: 867–888.

Magee, D.J. 1987. *Orthopedic physical assessment.* Philadelphia: WB Saunders Co: 170–174.

Malter, A.D., B. McNeney, J.D. Loeser, and R.A. Deyo. 1998. 5-year reoperation rates after different types of lumbar spine surgery. *Spine* 23: 814–20.

Manniche, C., H.F. Skall, L. Braendholt, B.H. Christensen, L. Christophersen, B. Ellegaard, A. Heilbuth, M. Ingerslev, O.E. Jorgensen, E. Larsen, L. Lorentzen, L., C.J. Nielsen, H.N. Nielsen, and M. Windelin. 1993. Clinical trial of postoperative dynamic back exercises after first lumbar discectomy. *Spine* 18: 92–7.

Mayer, T., M.J. McMahon, R.J. Gatchel, B. Sparks, A. Wright, and P. Pegues. 1998. Socioeconomic outcomes of combined spine surgery and functional restoration in workers' compensation spinal disorders with matched controls. *Spine* 23: 598–606.

McFarland, C. 1994. Considerations for physical therapy management of the postoperative spine patient. *Orthopaedic Physical Therapy Practice* 6: 8–11.

McKenzie, R.A. 1991. *The lumbar spine: Mechanical diagnosis and treatment.* New Zealand: Spinal Publications: 27–48.

Moffroid, M.T., L.D. Haugh, A.J. Haig, S.M. Henry, and M.H. Pope. 1993. Endurance training of trunk extensor muscles. *Phys Ther* 73: 3–10.

Morgan D. 1988. Concepts in functional training and postural stabilization for the low back injured. *Top Acute Care Trauma Rehabil* 2: 8–17.

Nelson, B.W., D.M. Carpenter, T.E. Dreisinger, M. Mitchell, C.E. Kelly, and J.A. Wegner 1999. Can spinal surgery be prevented by aggressive strengthening exercise? A prospective study of cervical and lumbar patients. *Arch Phys Med Rehabil* 80: 20–25.

Nykvist, F., M. Hurme, H. Alaranta, M. Kaitsaari. 1995. Severe sciatica: a 13-year follow-up of 342 patients. *Eur Spine J* 4: 335–8.

Oratec Interventions, Inc. 1999. Intradiscal ElectroThermal (tm) (IDET tm) Therapy: Physician's guide to post-procedural care. Oratec, Menlo Park, CA.

O'Sullivan, P.B., L.T. Twoomey, and G.T. Allison. 1997. Evaluation of specific stabilizing exercise in the treatment of chronic low back pain with radiologic diagnosis of spondylosis or spondylolisthesis. *Spine* 22: 2959–2967.

Paris, S.P. 1985. Physical signs of instability. *Spine* 10: 277–279.

Paris, Stanley P. 1998. "Whole spine stabilization." Course presented at Texas Physical Therapy Association Annual Conference.

Poole, Russell. 1997. "Postoperative management of mechanical disorders of the spine." Course presented by the McKenzie Institute in Dallas, Texas.

Potvin, J.R., and P.R. O'Brien. 1998. Trunk muscle co-contraction increases during fatiguing isometric lateral bend exertions. Possible indications for spine stabilization. *Spine* 23: 774–781.

Richardson, C., G. Jull, P. Hodges, and J. Hides. 1999. *Therapeutic exercise for spinal segmental stabilization in low back pain.* London: Churchill Livingstone.

Richardson, J.K., and Z.A. Iglarsh. 1994. *Clinical orthopaedic physical therapy.* Philadelphia: W.B. Saunders Company, 137–138.

Robinson, R. 1991. The new back school prescription: stabilization training, Part I. *Spine: State of the art reviews;* 5: 341–355.

Rothman, R.H., and F.A. Simeone. 1992. *The Spine Volume I, Third edition.* Philadelphia: W.B. Saunders Company.

Routhaupt, D., T. Laser, H. Ziegler, and K. Liebig. 1997. [Orthopedic hippotherapy in postoperative rehabilitation of lumbar intervertebral disk patients. A prospective randomized therapy study.] *Sportverletz Sportschaden* 11:63–69.

Saal, J.A. 1991. The new back school prescription: Stabilization training Part II. *Spine: State of the art reviews;* 5: 357–366.

_____. 1992. The new back school prescription: Stabilization training Part II. *Occupational medicine: State of the art reviews* 7: 40.

Saal, J.A., and J.S. Saal. 1989. Nonoperative treatment of herniated lumbar intervertebral disc with radiculopathy: An outcome study. *Spine* 14: 431–437.

Saunders, H.D. 1994. *Evaluation, treatment, and prevention of musculoskeletal disorders.* Minnesota: The Saunders Group.

Silcox, D.H., T. Daftari, S. Boden, S et al. 1995. The effect of nicotine on spinal fusion. *Spine* 20: 1549–1553.

Silhoven, T., K.A. Lindgren, O. Airaksinen, and H. Manninen. 1997. Movement disturbances of the lumbar spine and abnormal back muscle electromyographic findings in recurrent low back pain. *Spine* 22: 289–95.

Skinner, J.S. 1993. *Exercise testing and exercise prescription for special cases: Theoretical basis and clinical application,* 2nd edition. Philadelphia: Lea & Febiger.

Spine Care Associates of Tyler. 1994. The first six weeks (video).

Sullivan, J.G.B. 1992. The anesthesiologist's approach to back pain. In Rothman, R.H. & F.A. Simeone (eds). *The Spine, 3rd edition, Vol. II.* Philadelphia: W.B. Saunders Company: 1953–6.

Sutton, J.P., G. DeJong, and D. Wilkerson. 1996. Function-based payment model for inpatient medical rehabilitation: An evaluation. *Arch Phys Med Rehabil* 77: 693–701.

Taylor, V.M., R.A. Deyo, M. Ciol, and W. Kreuter. 1996. Surgical treatment of patients with back problems covered by workers' compensation vs. those with other sources of payment. *Spine* 21: 2255–9.

Waddell, G., J.A. McCulloch, E. Kimmel, and R.M. Venner. 1980. Nonorganic physical signs in low-back pain. *Spine* 5: 117–125.

Yoganandan, N., F. Pintar, D.J. Maiman, J. Reinartz, A. Sances, A.J. Larson, and J.F. Cusick. 1993. Kinematics of the lumbar spine following pedicle screw plate fixation. *Spine* 18: 504–12.

Annotated Bibliography

References on rehabilitation techniques and help with program design for spine patients. Texts with information on spine surgeries.

Alon, G., A. Dar, D. Katz-Behiri, D. Dahan, H.Z. Weingarden and R. Nathan. 1997. Survivors of CVA and head injury can improve selected impairments and functional measures following training with the NESS NMES system. *Phys Ther* 77: S84.

This is one of Dr. Alon's studies showing functional changes following specific regimens with electrical stimulation. His ideas are often helpful in identifying facilitation techniques in any patient with functional loss.

Alon, G., S.A. McCombe, S. Koutsantonis, et al. 1987. Comparisons of effects of electrical stimulation and exercise on abdominal musculature. *J Orthop Sports Phys Ther* 8: 567–573.

This study showed the greatest effect on muscle performance with a combination of the electrical stimulation and volitional exercise. The surprising result was that the next best group was electrical stimulation alone, and exercise alone came in last.

American College of Sports Medicine (ACSM). *Guidelines for exercise testing and prescription, 5th edition.* Baltimore: Williams & Wilkins, 1995.

A sixth edition is now available. This is a wonderful resource which can help you have standard parameters for allowing or not allowing exercise testing in individual patients.

Basmajian, J. and R. Nyberg. 1993. *Rational manual therapies.* Baltimore: Williams and Wilkins.

Includes almost every school of thought on manual therapy, and defines several terms which are often used loosely in orthopedics.

Bradford, D.S. (ed). 1997. *Master techniques in orthopedic surgery: The Spine.* Philadelphia: Lippincott-Raven.

Very complete explanations and excellent illustrations, photos, and study examples of many types of spine surgery. Includes fusions with some of the newer instrumentation: cervical and thoracic procedures. Some of the surgeons also discuss their problem-solving methods in diagnosing their patients and identifying those patients needing a particular surgery.

Elvey, R.L. 1986. The investigation of arm pain. In *Modern manual therapy,* edited by G.P. Grieve. New York: Churchhill Livingstone. 530–535.

Glasgow, E.F., L.T. Twomey, E.R. Scull, A.M. Kleynhans, R.M. Idczak (editors). 1985. *Aspects of Manipulative Therapy, 2nd edition.* New York: Churchill Livingstone.

Some big names in spines: Bogduk, Maitland, Wyke, Janda, and others have contributed chapters to this diverse and very thought-provoking book.

Greenman, P.E. 1996. *Principles of Manual Medicine, 2nd edition.* Baltimore: Williams & Wilkins.

This is another classic text that is very useful for reference regarding your technique for evaluation and treatment. It is a "verification check" essential for best practice.

Lindsay, K.W., and I. Bone. 1998. *Neurology and Neurosurgery Illustrated, 3rd edition.* New York: Churchill and Livingstone.

Excellent text with illustrations of instrumented and noninstrumented diagnostic tests, as well as signs and symptoms of many pathologies.

McKenzie, R.A. 1991. *The lumbar spine: Mechanical diagnosis and therapy.* New Zealand: Spinal Publications.

This is McKenzie's classic text which now has several controlled research studies backing much of his theory and method.

Mennell, J.M. 1992. *The musculoskeletal system: Differential diagnosis from symptoms and physical signs.* Gaithersburg, MD: Aspen Publishers Inc.
Three excellent chapters:
Ch. 6 Intricacies and interrelationships in the body systems;
Ch. 7 Cross-matching structure and pathologic changes in differential diagnosis of common causes of shoulder pain;
Ch. 8 Management of musculoskeletal pain.

Morgan, D. 1988. Concepts in functional training and postural stabilization for the low back injured. *Top Acute Care Trauma Rehabil* 2: 8–17.
One of the basic articles provided by Beverly Biondi in her introductory spine stabilization courses in the early 1990s.

Paris, S. 1985. Physical signs of instability. *Spine* 10: 277–9.

Paris, S. 1998. Stabilization. Whole spine stabilization. Course Notes.
A very worthwhile short course with additional views on stabilization, as usual, from Stanley Paris!

Porterfield, J., and C. DeRosa 1991. *Mechanical low back pain: Perspectives in functional anatomy.* W.B. Saunders Company.
Excellent anatomical illustrations. Complete explanations of several assessment and treatment techniques, and good supporting rationale for treatment choices. They also have an excellent text on the cervical spine with a similar title.

Robinson, R. 1991. The new back school prescription: stabilization training, Part I. *Spine: State of the art reviews* 5: 341–355.

Richardson, C., G. Jull, P. Hodges, and J. Hides. 1999. *Therapeutic exercise for spinal segmental stabilization in low back pain: Scientific basis and clinical approach.* London: Churchill Livingstone.

The second part of the title tells the reader about the value of this book. Evidence-based, but clinically-oriented, this book is valuable for the spine practitioner.

Saal, J.A. 1991. The new back school prescription: stabilization training, Part II. *Spine: State of the Art Reviews* 5: 357–366.

STUDIES DEALING WITH SPINE SURGERY OR USED FOR BACKGROUND IN THESE PROTOCOLS.

Atlas, S.J., R.A. Deyo, R.B. Keller, A.M. Chapin, D.L. Patrick, J.M. Long, and D.E. Singer. 1996. The Maine lumbar spine study, part II: 1-year outcomes of surgical and nonsurgical management of sciatica. *Spine* 21: 1777–1786.

This study involved 507 patients treated for sciatica, 275 surgical, and 232 nonsurgical. The study concluded with its one year follow-up that lumbar disc surgery provided a greater chance for rapid relief of symptoms. It reported more gradual relief without surgery.

_____. 1996. The Maine lumbar spine study, part III: 1-year outcomes of surgical and nonsurgical management of lumbar spinal stenosis. *Spine* 21: 1787–94.

Atlas, S.J., R.A. Deyo, D.L. Patrick, K. Convery, R.B. Keller, and D.E. Singer. 1996. The Quebec Task Force classification for spinal disorders and the severity, treatment, and outcomes of sciatica and lumbar spinal stenosis. *Spine* 21: 2885–92.

Used 1987 classification for 516 patients and found classification "strongly associated with the likelihood of having surgery".

BACKLetter. 1996. Hagerstown, MD: Lippincott-Raven Publishers.

Refers to the issue reporting the Faas study, and perhaps inaccurately entitled "Can exercise survive as a treatment for low back pain in the cost conscious world of managed care?" The Faas study reported on exercise for *acute* low back pain.

Brennan, G.P., B.B. Shulz, R.S. Hood, J.C. Zahniser, S.C. Johnson, and A.H. Gerber. 1994. The effects of aerobic exercise after lumbar microdiscectomy. *Spine* 19: 735–9.

Oxygen consumption was more than 3 times as important as any other single variable in differentiating between successful and nonsuccessful outcomes.

Carragee, E.J., E. Helms, and G.S. O'Sullivan. 1996. Are postoperative activity restrictions necessary after posterior lumbar discectomy? A prospective study of outcomes in 50 consecutive cases. *Spine* 21: 1893–7.

Patients had good outcomes without postoperative restrictions and with early return to activity.

Cherkin, D.C., R.A. Deyo, J.H. Street, and L. Barlow. 1996. Predicting poor outcomes for back pain seen in primary care using patients' own criteria. *Spine* 21: 2900–7.

Looks at errors in early intervention for low back pain that may be a part of the development of chronic spine problems.

Curtis, L., T. Mayer, and R. Gatchel. 1994. Physical progress and residual impairment quantification after functional restoration. *Spine* 19: 401–5.

Found identical increases in performance in nonsurgical and surgical patients following their intensive rehabilitation program.

DeLitto, A., M.T. Cibulka, R. Erhard, R.W. Bowling, and J.A. Tenhula. 1993. Evidence for use of an extension-mobilization category in acute low back pain syndrome; a prescriptive validation study. *Phys Ther* 73:216–23.

Proposed classification system for low back pain based on responses to mechanical treatments.

Deyo, R.A., and W.R. Phillips. 1996. Low back pain. A primary care challenge. *Spine* 21: 2826–32.

Deyo points out the lack of consistency in care for back pain, and shortcomings in the literature regarding outcomes for various treatment methods. Authors describe challenges for clinicians including: 1) better diagnostic strategies and classification of patients, 2) better theory explaining episodes of nonspecific low back pain, and 3) more methodological rigor for research on LBP.

Faas, A. 1996. Exercises: Which ones are worth trying, for which patients, and when? *Spine* 21: 2874–9.

Hides, J.A., C.A. Richardson, and G.A. Jull. 1996. Multifidus muscle recovery is not automatic after resolution of acute, first-episode low back pain. *Spine* 21: 2763–2769

Makes the case that lack of localized muscle support may be related to the high recurrence rate of low back pain, and provides evidence for muscle atrophy postoperatively. Implications for treatment!

Hinkley B.S. and M.E. Jaremko. 1997. Effects of 360-degree lumbar fusion in a workers' compensation population. *Spine* 22: 312–323.

Study of eighty workers' compensation patients with ninety-one percent reporting a positive response following "360" fusion, with rehabilitation starting the day after surgery and extending twelve to twenty-four weeks.

Ibarra, V.L. 1997. Spine update: Clinical pathways. *Spine* 22: 352–357
Good article to help develop clinical pathways. All steps explained.

Jette, D.U., and A.M. Jette. 1997. Professional uncertainty and treatment choices by physical therapists. *Arch Phys Med Rehabil* 78: 1346–51.
Refers to therapists' treatment choice inconsistencies when dealing with spine disorders. Both authors are therapists and cite this area as one needing attention.

Malter, A.D., B. McNeney, J.D. Loeser, and R.A. Deyo. 1998. 5-year reoperation rates after different types of lumbar spine surgery. *Spine* 23: 814–20.
Washington state study of 6376 patients having surgery in 1988 with a five-year follow-up. Compares complications and reoperation rates between fusions and nonfusion. There was no difference in reoperation rate, but complications were eighteen percent for fusions, seven percent for nonfusions.

McFarland C. 1994. Considerations for physical therapy management of the postoperative spine patient. *Orthopaedic Physical Therapy Practice* 6: 8–11.
Outlines program for postoperative patients based on evaluation findings and considering each affected tissue.

Nelson, B.W., D.M. Carpenter, T.E. Dreisinger, M. Mitchell, C.E. Kelly, and J.A. Wegner. 1999. Can spinal surgery be prevented by aggressive strengthening exercise? A prospective study of cervical and lumbar patients. *Arch Phys Med Rehabil* 80: 20–25.
An article which was a New Year's gift to therapists working with spine patients!

O'Sullivan, P.B., L.T. Twoomey, and G.T. Allison. 1997. Evaluation of specific stabilizing exercise in the treatment of chronic low back pain with radiologic diagnosis of spondylolysis or spondylolisthesis. *Spine* 22: 2959–67.

Specific exercise involved training of deep abdominals and lumbar multifidus in various postures. This program produced more pain relief and decreased functional disability when compared to control group in "other conservative treatment program."

Potvin, J.R., and P.R. O'Brien. 1998. Trunk muscle co-contraction increases during fatiguing isometric, lateral bend exertions: Possible indications for spine stabilization. *Spine* 23: 774–781.

Article helping support rationale for exercise selection.

Saal, J.S., J.A. Saal, and E.F. Yurth. 1996. Nonoperative management of herniated cervical intervertebral disc with radiculopathy. *Spine* 21: 1877–83.

Positive outcomes with an aggressive conservative care program for cervical HNP including traction and vigorous exercise.

Silhoven, T., K.A. Lindgren, O. Airaksinen, and H Manninen. 1997. Movement disturbances of the lumbar spine and abnormal back muscle electromyographic findings in recurrent low back pain. *Spine* 22: 289–95.

Motor control considerations in treatment program selection.

Yoganandan, N., F. Pintar, D.J. Maiman, J. Reinartz, A. Sances, A.J. Larson, and J.F. Cusick. 1993. Kinematics of the lumbar spine following pedicle screw plate fixation. *Spine* 18: 504–12.

Index